Net Gain

Table of Contents

Foreword

In view of the increasing intractability of malaria over the past decade, a great deal of activity and significant resources have been invested in research designed to develop and evaluate the impact of tools to reduce the disease burden in terms of morbidity and mortality in the population. Two attempts directed at prevention stand out: vaccines and insecticide-impregnated mosquito nets and other materials, such as curtains. Results of the first mortality study of insecticide-impregnated mosquito nets in The Gambia showed a reduction in all-cause mortality of 63% in children under 5 years of age (Alonso et al. 1991). These results led directly to the implementation of the National Impregnated Bednet Programme (NIBP) in The Gambia. The evaluation of NIBP confirmed the earlier study results showing a reduction in mortality of 25–38% in children under 5 in the context of a fully operational program (d'Alessandro et al. 1995).

The UNDP/World Bank/WHO Special Programme for Research and Training in Tropical Diseases (TDR), Canada's International Development Research Centre (IDRC), and other participating donors have sponsored three additional large-scale trials (populations of 60 000–120 000 each) in Africa to determine whether impregnated mosquito nets or curtains can reduce mortality in different epidemiological settings. The results of this research are critical to the formulation of policy recommendations regarding the use of insecticide-treated nets (ITNs) on a larger scale. Three of these trials (northern Ghana, coastal Kenya, and The Gambia) are now completed, and their results have been recently published.

There is now a need for operational research on the cost, feasibility, effectiveness, and long-term sustainability of this approach to define the role of ITNs at the national, district, and community levels in countries where the disease is endemic.

A joint TDR–IDRC initiative, currently under way, will attempt to solicit proposals and fund the required operational research over the next few years. The organization of an international meeting in Tanzania and the release of this book are the first steps in the process. For TDR and IDRC, the initiative demonstrates our continuing commitment to the development, promotion, and implementation of cost-effective interventions that will reduce the burden of tropical diseases in developing countries.

Maureen Law
Director General
Health Sciences Division
International Development
    Research Centre
Ottawa

Tore Godal
Director
UNDP/World Bank/WHO Special
    Programme for Research and
    Training in Tropical Diseases
Geneva

Acknowledgments

This work was supported in part by a grant from the Canadian International Development Agency. We are indebted to Professor W. Kilama, Director-General, National Institute for Medical Research, Tanzania, and his staff for hosting the IDRC–TDR workshop held in Dar es Salaam (Tanzania) in November 1994. C. Lengeler is supported by a grant from the Overseas Development Administration of the United Kingdom.

The author of Chapter 2 is grateful to Chris Curtis for his practical help in preparing this review and to Jane Miller, Mike Harrison, Tristan Nokes, Rachel Feilden, Susan Zimicki, Graham White, John Invest, Japhet Minjas, Susy Foster, Dominic Mlula, Rene, and many others who contributed views and ideas.

The author of Chapter 3 would like to thank all who responded to requests for information, especially Peter Evans, Tim Freeman, Jenny Hill, Axel Kroeger, Omer Mensah, Jos Miesen, Katie Reed, Mark Rowland, Clive Shiff, Eliab Some, and Susan Zimicki. Thanks also go to Chris Curtis and Anne Mills for comments on earlier drafts. Finally, many thanks to Jo Lines for technical support in preparing this review.

The author of Chapter 4 would like to thank all who shared reports and took time to discuss their projects, especially Tim Freeman, Susan Howard, Bill Brieger, Ane Haaland, Charles Oliver, Dennis Carroll, Camille Saade, Selim Rashed, John Berman, Jean-Paul Clark, Jim Sonneman, Deborah MacFarland, Andy Arata, Clive Schiff, Charles Delacollette, Jenny Hill, John Lenox, and Bob Hornik.

Executive Summary

Insecticide-treated nets (ITNs) have emerged in recent years as a promising tool to stem the rising tide of malaria in the world. Strong, convincing evidence is now available to document the beneficial impact of ITNs on malaria disease episodes in children.

Large studies in The Gambia, Ghana, and Kenya have documented a 17–63% reduction in overall child mortality as a result of ITN use. Several more ITN trials currently under way in Africa and elsewhere in the world, are confirming this efficacy in settings where malaria is highly endemic. Collectively, these studies reveal the potential of ITNs as an important public-health intervention in the limited arsenal of malaria-control strategies.

However, the cost, effectiveness, long-term sustainability, and practical feasibility of routine ("nonresearch") ITN-implementation programs are not yet well documented. The considerable impact measured in highly controlled trials has partly obscured the fact that ITN programs are both complex and costly. They will not be easy to implement and sustain on a large scale in routine health-intervention programing. Therefore, to better inform program managers on the "how to" of this intervention, more operational experience is needed. Novel approaches to the financing, distribution, periodic reimpregnation, and promotion of ITNs need to be explored.

Both the UNDP/World Bank/WHO Special Programme for Research and Training in Tropical Diseases (TDR) and Canada's International Development Research Centre (IDRC) believe that the ongoing efficacy research must now be matched with a comparable effort in effectiveness research. This is usually obtained through operational research done as much as possible with collaboration among researchers, implementing agencies (governmental and nongovernmental), and the private sector. TDR and IDRC have taken the initiative in this area, as outlined in Chapter 1, which also introduces ITNs as a malaria-control tool.

As a first step in the IDRC–TDR initiative, the available experience on technological, implementation, and promotional aspects of ITN trials and programs in Africa was reviewed (Chapters 2–4). These reviews attempt to cover all published documents and to identify unpublished reports ("gray literature"). The second step, based on these reviews, was an international workshop held in Dar es Salaam (Tanzania) in November 1994. It brought together researchers and implementors with the main objective to develop a strategic agenda for operational research. A summary of the main recommendations from this workshop are presented in Chapter 5.

ITN Technology

High-priority topics for research in the field of ITN technology are as follows:

- ❖ Standardize current field tests and develop new field tests to improve monitoring of mosquitoes' resistance to pyrethroids;
- ❖ Increase knowledge of interaction between insecticides and netting and of optimal insecticide doses;
- ❖ Develop a simple way to measure the dose of pyrethroids on netting;
- ❖ Develop new materials and procedures to reduce the need for retreating netting; and
- ❖ Improve packaging for insecticides.

ITN Implementation

Participants recommended systematic study of implementation models based on local variables such as actors, institutions, infrastructure, resources, and political conditions. Models could be "pure" (that is, completely private, governmental, social marketing, or nongovernmental) or "mixed" (that is, combining two or more types). Local- or national-level decision-support models and policy mapping were seen as tools worthy of development. In addition, essential work was recommended in areas with potential for significant improvement in future ITN programs:

- ❖ Studying the integration of ITN activities with other health interventions;
- ❖ Studying traditional and innovative financing mechanisms;
- ❖ Describing the effect of tax incentives for import, production, and sale of nets and insecticides; and
- ❖ Developing essential indicators for monitoring ITN programs.

ITN Promotion

Participants identified three areas where research in ITN promotion is needed:

* ❖ Acquiring nets or curtains;
* ❖ Using ITNs correctly; and
* ❖ Re-treating ITNs with insecticide correctly.

Defining the products, target audiences, key messages, and most cost-effective communication channels within given implementation models was seen as essential. With the aid of focused ethnographic research, promotional messages can be based on reinforcing and inhibiting beliefs in target populations. Participants also thought it important to study whether people are more motivated to acquire and use ITNs by perceived reductions in nuisance biting or by perceived reductions in disease. Another issue requiring investigation is optimal pricing of ITNs.

Several general recommendations were offered for political action to improve conditions for malaria control in general and ITN interventions in particular. Specifically, governments in countries where malaria is endemic are advised to consider ITNs as public-health goods and to help reduce their price by lifting taxes and duties on nets and public-health insecticides. In addition, governments should issue guidelines regarding the importation and safe use of insecticides. Bilateral and multilateral donor agencies are advised to assist national programs with standardized technical advice and, where appropriate, procurement support.

Chapter 1

From Research to Implementation

C. Lengeler, D. de Savigny, and J. Cattani

Malaria is one of the leading causes of morbidity and mortality in the developing world. Two billion people, or about 40% of the world's population, live in the 90 countries at risk (WHO 1994) (Figure 1). Global estimates of the malaria disease burden for 1992 indicated at least 300–500 million clinical cases annually, 90% of them in sub-Saharan Africa. Moreover, every year, malaria is associated with 1.5–2.7 million deaths, an overwhelming proportion of them in Africa (WHO 1994). In Africa, the malaria parasite, *Plasmodium falciparum*, accounts for about 25% of all childhood mortality below 5 years of age, excluding neonatal mortality (WHO 1994). Recent studies suggest that the percentage might actually be higher (Alonso et al. 1991; Kuate Defo 1995). The World Bank and the World Health Organization (WHO) rank malaria as the first cause of (disability-adjusted) life-year loss in Africa (World Bank 1993) and calculate an annual loss of 35 million future life–years from disability and premature mortality. Not only is malaria the largest single component of the disease burden in Africa, it is also a growing component as chemotherapy becomes less effective and alternative drugs become more expensive.

A Global Strategy for Malaria Control

In 1992, WHO convened a Ministerial Conference on Malaria in Amsterdam to define a Global Strategy for Malaria Control and stimulate new efforts to control malaria around the world (see Box 1). The four basic elements of the global strategy were defined as follows:

❖ Early diagnosis and prompt treatment;

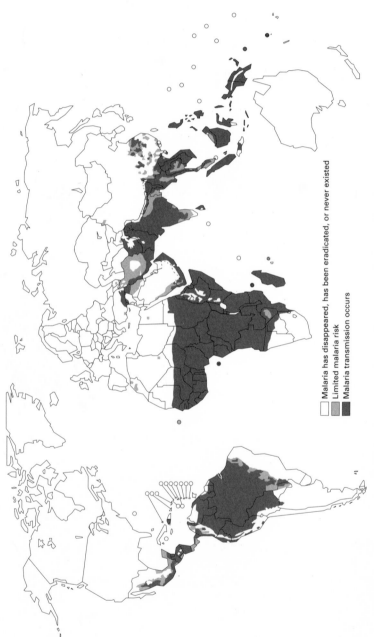

Figure 1. Malaria endemicity in the world (based on data from WHO 1994).

Malaria has disappeared, has been eradicated, or never existed
Limited malaria risk
Malaria transmission occurs

❖ Implementation of selective, sustainable, preventive measures, including vector control;

❖ Early detection, containment, and prevention of epidemics; and

❖ Fostering regular assessment of affected countries' malaria situation, especially the ecological, social, and economic determinants of the disease, by strengthening local capacities for basic and applied research.

This book specifically addresses the second element of the Global Strategy. Among preventive measures, one has emerged during the last decade as especially suitable for promotion in a primary health-care (PHC) approach: the use of insecticide-treated mosquito nets (ITNs). This approach has the potential to make a substantial difference to malaria control in areas where the disease is endemic, especially in Africa. The present initiative is largely concerned with applied research aspects at the local, national, and international levels and encourages partnership between researchers, implementors, and communities.

Box 1

The spirit of the Global Strategy for Malaria Control

The Global Strategy for Malaria Control calls for rational use of existing and future tools to control malaria. It recognizes that malaria problems vary enormously from epidemiological, ecological, social, and operational viewpoints and that sustainable, cost-effective control must therefore be based on local analysis. Based on decades of lessons from practice, the strategy is firmly rooted in the primary health-care approach and calls for the strengthening of local and national capabilities for disease control; for community partnership and the decentralization of decision-making; and for the integration of malaria-control activities with related disease-control programs and with other sectors, especially those concerned with education, agriculture, social development, and the environment. The stategy emphasizes the vital importance of continuing malaria research, locally and internationally, and of international teamwork in both control and research.

Source: WHO (1993b)

Early diagnosis and prompt treatment are still the basic elements of malaria control (WHO 1993a). Especially in young children, averting severe illness and death by timely treatment of every clinical episode with the correct dose of an effective drug is a most important way to reduce the burden imposed by malaria. Unfortunately, over the last 20 years, efforts to improve the situation have been hampered in many parts of the world by increasingly drug-resistant malaria parasites and insufficiently developed and financed public-health services. Enhancing integrated approaches to pediatric case management (such as the "integrated management of the sick child") must become a high priority for health ministries in countries where malaria is endemic.

Preventive measures, such as modifying the environment and spraying DDT and other insecticides indoors have worked in specific areas, including southern Africa (Zimbabwe, Botswana, and South Africa). Other countries have used these methods to reduce malaria significantly (for example, India, Sri Lanka, and Brazil) or to eliminate it (for example, the United States, Italy, Korea, several former Soviet republics, and many Caribbean islands). However, these achievements resulted from large disease-specific control programs and widespread, costly effort. Elimination of malaria has been achieved only in relatively wealthy countries, concurrent with major socioeconomic development. Moreover, transmission has been sustainably reduced only in countries where malaria is hypoendemic to mesoendemic (see Box 2).

Few malaria-prevention programs have been implemented or even considered in areas of Africa where the disease is hyperendemic to holoendemic. In these areas, roughly between latitudes 15°N and 20°S, transmission is intense and stable. Clinical disease and mortality are concentrated in young children; adolescents and adults have acquired enough immunity to survive recurrent infections. The few indoor-spraying programs undertaken since the 1960s were usually restricted to large cities where malaria transmission was low but nuisance biting intense. However, pilot house-spraying projects in Nigeria (Molineaux and Gramiccia 1980) and East Africa (Bradley 1991) demonstrated that such programs can reduce morbidity and mortality significantly.

Effective control programs are rare in areas of highest risk of malaria for economic, structural, and technical reasons. These areas lack the human, financial, and administrative resources required to carry out control programs in the traditional vertical form. As a result, hundreds of millions of people continue to be exposed to malaria (Figure 2) and

Box 2

Levels of malaria endemicity

Hypoendemic: Little transmission; malaria does not affect the general population importantly (spleen rate in children aged 2–9 years is less than 10%).

Mesoendemic: Typically found in rural communities with varying intensity of transmission (spleen rate in children is 11–50%).

Hyperendemic: Areas with intense but seasonal transmission where immunity is insufficient to prevent effects of malaria in all age groups (spleen rate in children constantly more than 50% and in adults, more than 25%).

Holoendemic: Areas with perennial high-degree transmission producing considerable immunity in all age groups, particularly adults (spleen rate in children constantly more than 75%, but low spleen rate in adults).

Source: Gilles (1993)

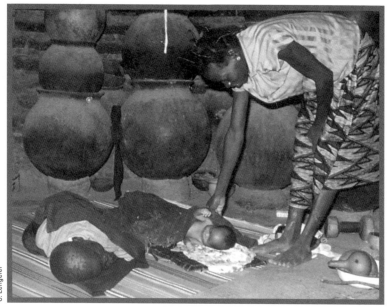

C. Lengeler

Figure 2. Children sleeping unprotected against malaria vectors.

the potential for lower mortality among children under 5 years of age has not been fulfilled.

For the first time, in ITNs, we have a malaria-prevention method so simple and safe that it can be organized and conducted locally by non-specialists.

Insecticide-Treated Nets

Most ITN trials and programs have used mosquito nets (also called bed-nets or nets). In some situations, however, nets are not practical, and curtains covering windows, doors, and eaves are preferred (see Chapter 2). For discussion purposes, ITNs and insecticide-treated curtains should be considered synonymous, and we use the term "nets" to refer to both. To eliminate the unfounded assumption that a bed is required for correct ITN use, we prefer to say "net" rather than "bednet."

To refer to applying insecticide to nets, authors use the terms "net impregnation," "net treatment," and "net dipping." Although net dipping refers to a specific way of applying insecticide to nets, these terms are essentially equivalent, and we use them interchangeably.

Applying residual insecticide to fabrics to prevent vector-borne diseases such as malaria and leishmaniasis began during World War II, when the Soviet, German, and US forces used insecticide-impregnated nets and clothing (Curtis et al. 1991). In the late 1970s, synthetic pyrethroids were found to be effective for this purpose — they are both highly insecticidal and of low toxicity to mammals.

Early ITN studies demonstrated the safety of pyrethroids and the significant impact of ITNs on various entomological parameters, such as the feeding success of the vector, vectorial capacity, and human-biting rates. These studies also helped define the action mechanism (repelling and killing) and optimal dosages for various combinations of netting and insecticide (see Chapter 2) (also reviewed in Rozendaal 1989; Carnevale et al. 1991; Curtis et al. 1991).

Impact of ITNs on malaria morbidity

A growing body of evidence suggests that ITN use substantially affects the frequency and severity of clinical episodes of malaria. More than 20 studies have been done in areas where malaria is endemic, including more than 12 in Africa. A systematic review of the evidence is beyond the scope of this publication, and interested readers should consult Curtis (1992a) and a review by Choi et al. (1995).

The epidemiologic design of ITN morbidity trials conducted in Africa was suboptimal, and their results should be interpreted cautiously. It is worth noting that most studies document a reduction of 20–63% (median, 45%) in malaria disease rates following introduction of ITNs. The results of standard clinical trials (randomized, controlled, and using sufficiently large samples) that measured impact on malaria disease in Africa are shown in Table 1. Other studies carried out in Mali (Ranque et al. 1984), Burkina Faso (Carnevale et al. 1988; Procacci et al. 1991), Tanzania (Lyimo et al. 1991; Stich et al. 1994), and Zaire (Karch et al. 1993) confirmed these results. Overall, ITNs' ability to reduce the number of disease episodes in communities with stable malaria is no longer questioned.

Impact of ITNs on malaria mortality

Given the major role of *P. falciparum* malaria as a direct and indirect cause of death in African children, the main public-health issue associated with ITNs is their effect on child mortality. Assessing the effect of an intervention on mortality requires very large, long-term, and therefore costly trials. In the first randomized, controlled trial of ITNs for mortality, Alonso et al. (1991) reported a 63% reduction in all mortality in children 1–4 years old.

Table 1. Impact of insecticide-treated mosquito nets (ITNs) on malaria morbidity in African children: an overview of selected trials.

Country	Transmission pressure[a]	Morbidity reduction (%) [b]	Source
The Gambia	1–10 (S)	45	Snow et al. (1987)
The Gambia	1–10 (S)	63	Snow, Lindsay et al. (1988)
Kenya	300 (P)	30	Sexton et al. (1990)
Kenya	300 (P)	40	Beach et al. (1993)
The Gambia	1–10 (S)	45	Alonso, Lindsay, Armstrong-Schellenberg, Keita et al. (1993)
Guinea Bissau	20–50 (S)	29	Jaenson et al. (1994)
Sierra Leone	20–40 (S)	49	Marbiah (1995)
Tanzania	300 (P)	55	Premji et al. (1995)
Kenya	10–30 (S)	44[c]	Nevill et al. (1996)

[a] Entomologic inoculation rate as infective bites per person per year, with seasonality indicated in parentheses: P, perennial; S, seasonal.
[b] Protective efficacy for uncomplicated malaria episodes (fever + parasitaemia), comparing children sleeping under ITNs with those who do not.
[c] Reduction in severe, life-threatening malaria.

The dramatic results of this first mortality trial prompted the UNDP/World Bank/WHO Special Programme for Research and Training in Tropical Diseases (TDR) to collaborate with many agencies to launch four large-scale trials to measure ITNs' effect on overall child mortality in various areas of Africa where malaria is endemic (Burkina Faso, The Gambia, Ghana, and Kenya). The agencies collaborating in this unique multicountry enterprise are listed in Figure 3.

These carefully randomized, controlled trials, covering a population of nearly 400 000, help define the potential benefits of ITN programs. Results of the three completed trials show a substantial reduction in child mortality, confirming ITN program benefits. An overview of the impact on child mortality is given in Table 2.

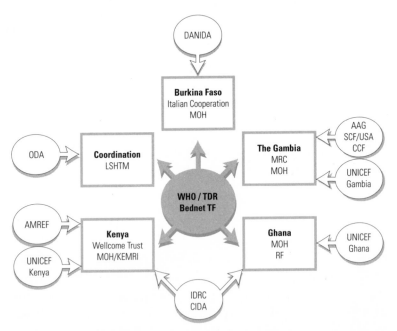

Figure 3. Agencies collaborating with the bednet Task Force (TF) of TDR on the four large-scale trials to measure the impact of ITNs on child mortality in Africa: the Canadian International Development Agency (CIDA), the International Development Research Centre (IDRC), the United Nations Children's Fund (UNICEF), the UK Overseas Development Agency (ODA), the Danish International Development Agency (DANIDA), the Wellcome Trust, the UK Medical Research Council (MRC), the African Medical Research Foundation (AMREF), the Italian Cooperation, the Rockefeller Foundation (RF), the London School of Hygiene and Tropical Medicine (LSHTM), Action Aid The Gambia (AAG), Save the Children Federation (SCF/USA), the Christian Children's Fund (CCF), the Kenyan Medical Research Institute (KEMRI), as well as various national ministries of health (MOHs).

Table 2. Impact of insecticide-treated mosquito nets on mortality in African children: an overview of published trials.

Country	Transmission pressure[a]	Coverage [c]	Mortality reduction[b] (%)	Source
The Gambia	1–10 (S)	High	63	Alonso et al. (1991)
The Gambia	1–10 (S)	Medium	25	d'Alessandro et al. (1995)
Kenya	10–30 (S)	High	33	Nevill et al. (1996)
Ghana	100–300 (S)	High	17	Binka et al. (1996)

[a] Entomologic inoculation rate as infective bites per person per year, with seasonality indicated in parentheses: S, seasonal.
[b] Protective efficacy against all causes of child mortality.
[c] Average net use by target group.

In 1996, the results of the fourth mortality trial (Burkina Faso) will be published. Further trials are planned for Kenya and Tanzania in areas of very high transmission pressure. It must be noted that the reduction in mortality from all causes seen in these trials exceeds the reduction predictable from current understanding of malaria-specific mortality rates. This finding emphasizes the underestimated contribution of malaria to child mortality in Africa (Snow et al. 1995) and the potentially large benefits of malaria-preventive interventions.

From Research Trials to Effective, Community-Based Interventions

The critical path: where are we now?

ITNs are now recognized as an efficacious intervention against malaria in all areas of Africa but those with the highest transmission pressure. However, the main lesson from earlier antimalaria efforts is that identifying an efficacious control tool is only one step toward an effective, sustainable malaria-control program (WHO 1993a). Most ITN mortality trials were implemented under strict control and with substantial financial, human, and technical resources — conditions hardly resembling those in which control programs must be delivered and sustained in PHC or other delivery and financing contexts. This raises the issues of feasibility and cost effectiveness of fully implementing ITN programs and of community-level sustainability and equitability over the long term.

The preceding brief overview of ITN morbidity and mortality trials reveals the growing body of evidence of the efficacy of ITN interventions in reducing overall mortality and malaria-specific disease among children. However, a distinction must be drawn between **efficacy**, which is determined in research field trials under excellent conditions of targeting, coverage, and compliance, and **effectiveness**, which, simply put, is the efficacy level achieved by the same intervention under real-life, program-delivery conditions (see Box 3).

Health researchers, donors, and program implementors often do not distinguish between efficacy and effectiveness. Therefore, they sometimes overestimate the validity of field-trial research results for programs at the national or international level. When randomized, controlled field trials indicate an efficacious new child-survival technology, it is tempting to implement broad-based policy immediately. However, direct transition from field trials to policy and national strategy skips an essential intermediate step in which researchers, program implementors, and donors collaborate in operational studies of more realistic intervention-delivery experiences.

Recently, there have been calls to base health intervention priorities and investments not only on costs or efficacy but also on cost-effectiveness (World Bank 1993). To generate these data, we must move beyond efficacy research to new partnerships for effectiveness research.

The path from efficacy research to effectiveness research is outlined very simply in Figure 4 (see also Curtis et al. 1991; Lengeler and Snow 1996). Starting in the early 1980s, much research was led by entomologists and focused on the efficacy of ITNs against malaria vectors.

Box 3

Efficacy and effectiveness

Efficacy: The extent to which a specific health intervention produces a beneficial result under ideal conditions. Efficacy should be determined from the results of a randomized, controlled trial.

Effectiveness: The extent to which a specific health intervention produces a beneficial result when deployed in the field under routine conditions.

Source: Based on Last (1995).

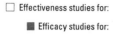

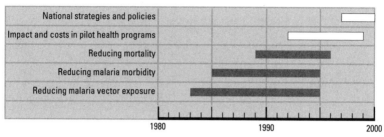

Figure 4. Stages of research on insecticide-treated nets.

Success at this permitted collaborative research between entomologists and malariologists on ITN efficacy for reducing malaria morbidity in the mid-1980s and for reducing child mortality from 1989 onward. In the mid-1990s we had compelling efficacy results for ITNs. Now it is time to move on to operational research on realistic regional-level ITN implementation programs.

Increasingly, donors and health ministries in countries where malaria is endemic are considering implementing ITN programs as integral components of national malaria-control strategies. However, implementing a large-scale malaria-prevention program based on ITNs is complex because substantial direct, indirect, and opportunity costs are involved, both for implementing agencies and for communities.

ITN trials have already produced much information on the managerial, human, and material elements important to successful implementation and use of ITNs. Some aspects have already been reviewed by Carnevale and Coosemans (1995). The second mortality trial conducted in The Gambia (d'Alessandro et al. 1995), which was actually more an effectiveness trial than an efficacy trial, also produced compelling data on cost effectiveness — it indicated that the cost for each death averted was $600[1] (Aikins 1995). Furthermore, several nonresearch ITN programs now running in Africa, Asia, and Latin America are producing much relevant operational experience in implementation, financing, and sustainability. Some of this evidence is published, but most is "gray" literature and therefore not widely available (Lengeler et al. 1996). Moreover, much of this experience has never been recorded formally. It is,

---

[1] Unless otherwise indicated, all monetary values are expressed in US currency.

therefore, important to disseminate this information and identify knowledge gaps. Much experience from more routine and realistic ITN programs must still be collected to optimize this malaria-control approach. Also, novel approaches to financing ITN programs, impregnating nets, and distributing ITNs have yet to be explored.

Where do we need to go?

TDR and IDRC are both convinced that the efficacy-research effort must be followed up with a comparable operational-research effort. This research would inform implementing agencies about the best options for implementing sustainable ITN programs. It should certainly be done as much as possible by collaborating researchers and implementing agencies (governmental, nongovernmental, and private-sector). Researchers, implementors, and donors should all benefit from this collaboration. At this stage of development, researchers must focus increasingly on the requirements of implementors, who may need support for increased monitoring and for testing new implementation approaches. Similarily, we hope that this initiative will encourage ITN implementors to undertake more systematic operational research on their programs.

The current initiative is a TDR–IDRC joint venture. Its general objective is to develop and promote a strategic agenda for operational research on ITNs to make them as cost effective and sustainable as possible in routine conditions.

Both TDR and IDRC will use this agenda to guide their support for malaria-control research efforts. Implementing agencies are encouraged to contribute to the agenda and to include operational research in their own programs.

The Canadian International Development Agency and IDRC already support related research in Africa designed to

❖ Test various community-level models of ITN delivery and financing;

❖ Explore the local potential for net manufacture;

❖ Describe markets for nets in countries where malaria is endemic;

❖ Review legislative changes, especially in taxation, most likely to improve access to nets and insecticide (PATH 1995); and

❖ Map malaria transmission risks pertinent to ITN program strategies.

How do we get there?

The TDR–IDRC initiative has **three stages**: comprehensive reviews of operational aspects of ITNs; an international workshop to look at specific research issues; and, finally, support of research proposals.

Review of operational aspects of ITNs

Most data on the operational aspects of ITNs are either unpublished or not widely available. Therefore, the first stage was to undertake comprehensive reviews of available information. The reviews addressed the following ITN issues:

❖ Intervention technology;

❖ Intervention implementation; and

❖ Intervention promotion.

In addition to the reviews, topics are outlined for further applications and research. Discussion at the international workshop was based on the reviews that produced chapters 2–4 of this book.

International workshop

Hosted by the Tanzanian National Institute of Medical Research (NIMR) in Dar es Salaam, Tanzania, the workshop was held 22–25 November 1994. It convened researchers conducting various types of ITN trials and workers involved either in ITN programs or donor agencies (see list of participants in Appendix 2). The two main objectives of this workshop were to

❖ Discuss, critique, and contribute to the three reviews; and

❖ Draw up an operational-research agenda for ITN interventions.

The meeting dealt mainly with specific research issues but also considered several more general recommendations for political action. The recommendations are detailed at the end of each review and are summarized in Chapter 5. The workshop acknowledged some confusion on the definition of operational research. Although the difference between operational research and program monitoring is not easy to define (see Box 4), this difficulty was not seen as a problem. The two concepts exist on the same practical continuum — and operational research usually must be done in the context of implementation programs.

Box 4

Operational research and program monitoring

Operational research: Systematic study, by observation or intervention, of the working of a system, such as a health service, with a view to improvement.

Program monitoring: Continuous oversight of the implementation of an intervention that seeks to ensure that input deliveries, work schedules, targeted outputs, and other required actions proceed according to plan.

Source: Based on Last (1995).

Eliciting and supporting operational research proposals

The third stage of the initiative began in mid-1995 with a call for proposals on the identified research priorities (Lengeler et al. 1996). TDR reviewed the first set of proposals in September 1995.

An initiative to facilitate ITN operational research

In the following chapters, significant efforts were made to review all available sources on ITN technology, implementation, and promotion. However, it is impossible either to perform a perfect retrospective review or to identify all unexplored issues and options. Some information is unavailable, and no general policy framework exists for ITNs.

For example, no one has adequately examined the option of distributing ITNs at little or no cost to high-risk groups, such as newborns and pregnant women, through established health-care channels, such as immunization and mother-and-child programs. This approach could not be recommended without careful consideration of cost effectiveness and the specific interests of program managers and donor agencies; no such program currently exists.

Even with such a well-defined intervention, operational research takes many forms and requires a wide range of skills. Both multi- and interdisciplinary in nature, it is highly collaborative. The challenge is great, but so are the rewards. Rarely do we encounter an intervention so efficacious at reducing child mortality in Africa. We must make every effort to make this promise a reality.

Chapter 2

The Technical Issues

J.D. Lines

Most people are familiar with the two elements of an insecticide-treated net (ITN). The idea of using a bednet is not new in the tropics, even in places where nets themselves are uncommon. Insecticides are also widely familiar, in one form or another. Agricultural chemicals are used in farming communities, mosquito coils are sold even in remote towns, and traditional plant products are used in many rural areas. The combination of net and insecticide is less familiar, even though it has a long history (Lindsay and Gibson 1988); for example, nets impregnated with DDT were used during World War II (Harper et al. 1947).

The use of pyrethroids on nets is new, however, and does have the promise of a new technology. To begin with, it gives outstandingly effective personal protection against nuisance insects. Indeed, users' enthusiasm suggests that this technology might eventually appear in shops beside the aerosol insecticides and mosquito coils. Moreover, the efficacy of pyrethroid-treated nets for malaria control in Africa has been confirmed by careful trials (for reviews, see Curtis 1992a; Choi et al. 1995). At last, we have a method of prevention that is comparable in epidemiological effect with house spraying, yet simple and safe enough for application by nonspecialists. ITNs may therefore permit what was previously impossible: truly effective community-based malaria control in Africa. The technology is so simple and the problem of malaria so severe that ITNs are a highly attractive public-health intervention.

To realize this promise, however, the technology must first be delivered to users. Public-health planners are now considering the structures and processes required to make treated nets available. Both public health systems and the commercial market could contribute, but it is not yet clear what roles each should take. Different distribution systems may be needed for nets and for insecticide. There are two reasons for this. First, nets are already available in many places, but the insecticide generally is not. Second, a net lasts several years and requires repeated re-treatment with insecticide. There is, therefore, little point in distributing treated nets unless an effective re-treatment system can also be established.

So far, China is the only country where a system for the routine treatment of large numbers of nets has been going on long enough to prove sustainable (Curtis 1992b; Xu et al. 1994; Cheng et al. 1995). Although the Chinese system is a useful model, it cannot be replicated in places where the primary health-care system is weak and few people have nets. Treated bednet and curtain projects outside China have used a range of approaches, but no consensus on the best strategy has emerged. Many successful technologies have to pass through an initial period of evolution and adaptation before a form eventually emerges that proves useful in a wide variety of circumstances. The technology of pyrethroid-impregnated nets and curtains has evolved little, and it is likely that this process has not yet really begun.

This review considers the technical aspects of treated nets, focusing on the range of materials available. The choice depends on efficacy, safety, and convenience. This chapter therefore begins by explaining how treated nets work and how efficacy can be compared. Safety and convenience can be judged only in context, so the people and organizations that may be involved are also considered. The chapter then deals with the materials and treatment processes.

Measures of Entomological Impact

ITNs affect mosquitoes in several ways (see Box 5), and this section discusses how to measure these impacts. Most of the useful comparative measures are entomological — many combinations of fabric and insecticide are possible, but only a few can be tested in epidemiological trials.

Insecticide deposit

Measuring the concentration of insecticide on an ITN is essential for quality control in routine operations. Currently, the only available methods are sophisticated and costly gas chromatography or high-pressure liquid chromatography tests (Hossain et al. 1989; Lindsay, Hossain et al. 1991). In most trials and pilot projects, only a few samples can be tested, and it is, therefore, impossible to measure patchiness of the deposit within a net or variability between nets. Moreover, test results are not returned

Box 5

How ITNs work

Ideally, an untreated net should provide a complete physical barrier to mosquitoes. In practice, even intact, tucked-in nets offer only partial protection; mosquitoes quickly find any body part touching the net or inadvertently left uncovered. Good protection generally requires a very high standard of care in maintenance as well as in use. A net with holes is better than no net at all, but unless the holes are small, it offers very little protection (Port and Boreham 1982; Charlwood 1986).

Pyrethroids are excito-repellent insecticides; their effects on insect behaviour include inhibition of feeding and driving insects from their hiding places. Pyrethroids share this property with DDT but not with other common public health insecticides. The presence of a pyrethroid on a net greatly reduces a mosquito's ability to feed through the fabric or penetrate small gaps in it (Curtis et al. 1991). An ITN with large holes protects as well as an intact untreated bednet, reducing biting by up to 95% (Lines et al. 1987; Lindsay, Hossain et al. 1991; Miller et al. 1991; Pleass et al. 1993; Curtis et al. 1992).

Personal protection against mosquitoes is an individual gain and is all that can be expected when an ITN is used in isolation. ITNs kill some of the mosquitoes that come to bite, however, and this can produce a bonus for the whole community. When many people in a village use ITNs, marked reductions have sometimes been seen not only in the density of the local mosquito population but also, and especially, in the sporozoite rate. This kind of "mass effect" does not always occur, but when it does, it benefits everyone in the village.

quickly enough to provide feedback for modifying procedures. One most pressing research need, therefore, is a test suitable for use in field laboratories. A simple test of presence or absence is better than nothing, and one such test has already been field tested in The Gambia (Muller et al. 1994). A quantitative test would be much better, and both chemical and serological possibilities are being explored (S.W. Lindsay, personal communication). A pigment added to insecticide to indicate presence and consistency might be helpful, especially if it faded at the same rate as the insecticide decayed.

Insecticidal action

ITNs are treated both to prevent mosquitoes from biting and to kill them. Protection against biting can be measured easily by pressing an arm against the fabric or by observing whether mosquitoes pass through holes or gaps (for example, Hossain and Curtis 1989; Jana-Kara et al. 1995).

A bioassay is the only test simple and quick enough for routine use with large numbers of ITNs (Lindsay, Hossain et al. 1991; Miller 1994a) and is the primary tool for comparing different types of net treatment (see Figure 6). A bioassay consists of confining mosquitoes in contact with the insecticide deposit and measuring their mortality. In routine operations, bioassays can be used to monitor treatment quality and, at 1- to 3-month intervals, to monitor the residual activity of the insecticide deposit.

Mosquitoes can be confined and exposed in various ways, and the outcome measure may be the median time required for mosquitoes to be knocked down or, more commonly, the proportion dead after a fixed exposure period (Rozendaal 1989; Njunwa et al. 1991). The main problem with current bioassay techniques is the variation that is usually observed between replicate tests. In consequence, many replications are needed to produce reliable results. Standardization of methods for maximizing repeatability is needed.

Experimental-hut trials

Even brief exposure to pyrethroids can change insects' behaviour in ways that affect the degree and pattern of further exposure (see Box 5). This interaction produces complex effects that cannot be measured by simple bioassays. Experimental huts are more realistic: the human bait is asleep, and the mosquitoes are free to enter, attempt to feed, and leave the hut. Special modifications to the hut (Smith and Webley 1969; Curtis et al. 1992) allow accurate sampling of mosquitoes that are driven outside, as well as those that are killed — this is impossible in ordinary rooms. In this way, several effects can be distinguished.

> ❖ *Deterrency*: Fewer mosquitoes enter the room. Pyrethroids are contact insecticides with a very low vapour pressure, so it is surprising that mosquitoes are affected at all before they enter the room. With ITNs treated less than 6 weeks previously, the vapour from the solvent itself may be deterrent (Lindsay, Adiamah 1991),

but an airborne effect from the pyrethroid is also evident (Somboon 1993). Smith and Webley (1969) worked with experimental huts sprayed with DDT, which also has a very low vapour pressure, and demonstrated similar airborne effects from insecticide-contaminated dust.

❖ *Feeding inhibition*: Of the mosquitoes that enter the room, fewer feed, which is particularly noticeable with ITNs with holes.

❖ *Mortality*: A proportion of female mosquitoes are killed by the insecticide, either before or after feeding.

❖ *Repellency:* Mosquitoes that would have stayed in the room to rest are stimulated to leave.

Treated curtains and nets that are large in relation to the room protect against biting mainly by deterring mosquitoes from entering the room. Smaller ITNs protect mostly by killing mosquitoes that have already entered the room or by driving them outside before they feed (Lines et al. 1987; Curtis et al. 1992).

Experimental-hut trials confirm bioassay measures of the duration of the residual efficacy of treated bednets, typically giving figures of 6 months (without washing) for permethrin at 200–500 mg/m^2 (Figure 5) and 12 months for lambdacyhalothrin and deltamethrin at 10–25 mg/m^2 (Lines et al. 1987; Curtis et al. 1991; Curtis 1992a; Curtis et al. 1994).

Most experimental-hut trials of ITNs were performed in Africa with *Anopheles gambiae* s.l. Satisfactory methods have yet to be developed for measuring how well ITNs protect someone sleeping outside or in a house with incomplete walls, such as are found in Latin America and Southeast Asia.

Experimental-hut trials measure feeding inhibition and killing at the individual level. They cannot indicate whether female mosquitoes driven outdoors feed elsewhere (for example, on unprotected people) or, if so, whether host choice is affected. Neither can the trials predict whether the proportion of mosquitoes killed would, with large-scale ITN use, amount to a mass effect on the local mosquito population (see Box 5). The balance between these two opposite effects (diversion and mass killing) determines whether the use of ITNs by some people is detrimental or beneficial to other people in the same community who do not have nets.

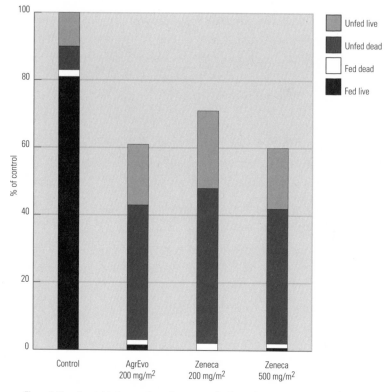

Figure 5. Experimental-hut comparison of nets treated with two formulations of permethrin with different *cis–trans* isomer ratios (AgrEvo 25:75; Zeneca 40:60), and of the latter at high and moderate dosages, after 5 months of routine domestic use (source: Curtis et al. 1994).

Mass effects

When ITNs are used consistently over a wide enough area against an anthropophilic vector (one that prefers to feed on human hosts), female mosquitoes risk death whenever they try to feed. In these circumstances, the density of the local mosquito population may drop, as may the parous rate and the sporozoite rate. Such effects were seen in village-scale ITN trials in Burkina Faso (Robert and Carnevale 1991), Tanzania (Magesa et al. 1991), Kenya (Beach et al. 1993), and Zaire (Karch et al. 1993). In Tanzania, the effects on density and sporozoite rate reduced the rate of infectious biting of unprotected people by more than 90 %. Detailed age-grading of mosquitoes showed that this was due to reduced survival (Magesa et al. 1991), presumably because of mosquito mortality. ITNs are unlikely to be repellent enough to drive mosquitoes from treated to untreated villages.

In the early village-scale trials in The Gambia, it was not clear whether or not there was a mass effect as well as improved personal protection. The effect on biting rates at the community level was estimated by catching and counting fed female mosquitoes in indoor-resting catches and in exit traps. Fewer fed female mosquitoes were collected in this way in untreated rooms in untreated villages than in treated rooms in treated villages (Snow, Lindsay et al. 1988; Lindsay, Snow, Broomfield et al. 1989). With a repellent treatment, however, the exophily induced in fed female mosquitoes can bias such estimates. This bias exists because exit traps catch a smaller fraction of the mosquitoes that leave a room than spray catches of those that stay.

In a later trial, sampling in treated villages was done in "sentinel" rooms without ITNs; no difference was observed between treated and untreated villages in the number of fed female mosquitoes collected in such rooms. Parous rates and sporozoite rates were also similar (Lindsay, Snow, Broomfield et al. 1989; Lindsay et al. 1993; M. Quinones and J. Lines, unpublished); in other words, there was no mass effect in The Gambia.

Thus, because of the repellency effect on fed female mosquitoes, indoor-resting catches in rooms with ITNs (for example, Jaenson et al. 1994) probably exaggerate the effect of ITNs on the village-level infective biting rate. It is not yet clear whether light-trap catches in rooms with ITNs are similarly biased. In general, when testing for a mass effect, sentinel sampling stations without ITNs are preferable in treated villages.

The vector species does not seem to be the reason why a mass effect has been seen in some African trials but not in others: *An. gambiae* s.s. is the main vector in both The Gambia and Tanzania. ITNs might kill fewer mosquitoes in The Gambia because of differences in fabric and treatment methods (Nagle 1994). Killing effects could also be masked in The Gambia by movement of mosquitoes between treated and untreated villages (M.C. Thomson and M. Quinones, personal communication).

Outside Africa, clear evidence of a mass effect with *An. minimus* was reported from Assam, India (Jana-Kara et al. 1995), but not from Thailand (Somboon 1993). The difference between these two cases seems to be related to mosquito behaviour: in Assam, *An. minimus* is still endophilic and anthropophilic, but it is now zoophilic and exophilic in Thailand (Ismail et al. 1978). Weaker evidence of a mass effect with *An. farauti* was reported from the Solomon Islands (Hii et al. 1993; Kere et al. 1993).

The possibility of a mass effect should be considered when planning the scale and coverage of ITN projects, because the community can benefit extensively. However, mass effects are improbable with zoophilic species and uncertain even with anthropophilic ones. Moreover, a mass effect is likely only if ITN use is almost universal in an area — and it is not even certain how large the area must be. Concerted community-wide ITN use may be more difficult to achieve than a gradual, household-by-household increase in coverage. Mass effects should, therefore, be regarded as an important additional benefit of a high rate of coverage and not as a factor that should be allowed to constrain other, more efficient distribution systems.

Diversion

When hungry mosquitoes are prevented by a net from feeding on one person, do they succeed in feeding on another host? How long does exposure to the insecticide continue to hamper a mosquito's subsequent efforts to obtain a blood meal? Like mass effects, diversion is relevant to distribution. If ITNs merely alter the bite distribution and do not reduce the number of bites, then ITN users may be protected only at others' expense.

There is little doubt that untreated nets divert mosquitoes to other hosts nearby. In Tanzania, Lines et al. (1987) estimated the amount of biting on two children sleeping in an experimental hut in three conditions: when a net was used by neither child, by one child, and by both children. When one child slept under an untreated net, the other received more bites. With the net treated with permethrin, however, the opposite effect was observed: the child without a net was bitten less than when both were unprotected.

Are mosquitoes diverted from treated to untreated houses? Lindsay et al. (1992) measured mosquito entry into six experimental huts: five occupied by sleepers with untreated nets and one occupied by a sleeper with an ITN. The rate of entry into the untreated huts was not affected by proximity to the ITN. This finding suggests that diverted mosquitoes do not concentrate in nearby houses but does not rule out the possibility that they disperse and then resume searching for a blood meal.

Village-scale studies in Papua New Guinea (Charlwood and Graves 1987) showed that ITNs can divert mosquitoes from humans to animals. After ITNs were introduced, the proportion of blood meals taken from animals increased and the proportion of blood meals taken from people decreased. Diversion to animals clearly benefits humans, but mosquitoes would presumably be diverted to other humans if fewer animal hosts were available and ITN coverage was incomplete. However, village-scale trials in Africa found no evidence of a decrease in the human blood index either in small samples of outdoor-resting female mosquitoes in Tanzania

(Magesa et al. 1991) or among indoor-resting female mosquitoes in The Gambia (Lindsay et al. 1993; M. Quinones and J. Lines, unpublished). When most people in a village begin using ITNs, the balance between the opposing effects of diversion and killing can be measured directly by counting the number of mosquitoes attempting to feed on unprotected humans outdoors or in rooms without ITNs. Biting rates have either declined or remained unchanged (Magesa et al. 1991; Robert and Carnevale 1991; Beach et al. 1993; Karch et al. 1993; Lindsay et al. 1993; Somboon 1993; Jana-Kara et al. 1995; M. Quinones and J. Lines, unpublished). Overall, the evidence suggests that acquisition of an ITN by one person tends to be either marginally beneficial or neutral to others — as long as the ITN remains treated.

Effects on the biting cycle

Two studies have reported effects on mosquitoes' daily biting cycle. In Papua New Guinea, Charlwood and Graves (1987) observed that when ITNs were introduced into a village, biting by *An. farauti* peaked earlier in the night (and the gonotrophic (oviposition) cycle lasted longer). Njau et al. (1993) observed a similar change in Tanzania when a village was divided into four groups of houses, three of which were provided with either untreated nets or ITNs treated with lambdacyhalothrin or deltamethrin. Biting peaked earlier in houses with ITNs but not in houses with untreated nets. In either case, such prompt effects are presumably temporary and phenotypic and must be contrasted with the permanent evolutionary changes in the biting cycle of the Solomon Islands mosquitoes of the *An. punctulatus* complex apparently caused by spraying DDT (Sloof 1964). Other trials, such as those in The Gambia (M. Quinones and J. Lines, unpublished) and Sierra Leone (E. Magbity and J. Lines, unpublished), have reported no biting-cycle changes.

The peak biting time of the local vector might be expected to be an important determinant of ITN effectiveness: ITNs are more likely to affect late biters than early biters. However, in Guatemala (Richards et al. 1993) and China (Li et al. 1989; Curtis 1992b; Cheng et al. 1995), where the main vector species are both early biters, malaria has been successfully controlled by ITNs. Further examples can be expected from trials in India, where the biting time of *An. culicifacies* s.l. varies geographically and between sibling species (T. Adak and V.P. Sharma, personal communication).

Resistance to pyrethroids

Resistance must be regarded as an unavoidable threat whenever an insecticide is used widely, intensely, and for extended periods. Unfortunately, pyrethroids are probably the only insecticides suitable for use on ITNs. Some argue that, as a public-health tool, pyrethroid ITNs are doomed from the start. The same can be said of any antibiotic or antimalarial drug, but no one would suggest that eventual resistance is a good reason not to use new drugs. There are equity implications, however. Genes for insecticide susceptibility in mosquito populations can be regarded as a finite resource that could be exhausted by people with easy access to ITNs before less-privileged people can benefit.

In some insects, for example, the day-biting mosquito *Aedes aegypti*, the commonest form of DDT resistance confers cross-resistance to pyrethroids. Fortunately, the same is apparently not true of *Anopheles*: all DDT resistance characterized so far in malaria vectors is caused by specific DDT-detoxification mechanisms. Pyrethroids have been widely used in agriculture, and there have been several reports of this causing resistance in various *Anopheles* species (Lines 1988; Roberts and Andre 1994; Kroeger et al. 1995). Such reports, however, are generally not well substantiated (Malcolm 1988); for example, they often lack evidence that the observed resistance is heritable.

Field-selected pyrethroid resistance in *Anopheles* has been well studied in only one case — that of *An. stephensi* in Dubai (Laddoni et al. 1990; Sivananthan et al. 1992). The resistance arose after pyrethroids were used as larvicides, but in the laboratory it also protects adult mosquitoes against ITNs (Curtis et al. 1993).

ITNs have been widely used over a long period only in parts of China, notably Sichuan, where neither resistance nor control failure have appeared (Curtis 1992b; Cheng et al. 1995). However, a moderate (2.5-fold) decrease in susceptibility to permethrin was reported from a local ITN trial in Kenya (Vulule et al. 1994). The significance of this decrease remains unclear. The data may indicate either a homogeneous increase in tolerance or the presence of a small proportion of highly resistant individuals. The latter would be more ominous, as it would suggest scope for further evolution.

Confirmed cases of pyrethroid resistance remain extremely rare in *Anopheles* species. To preserve susceptibility, selection for resistance should be minimized. Unfortunately, the only clear priorities for resistance management relate to research, not implementation (Taylor and Georghiou 1979; Curtis 1987; Tabashnik 1990; Curtis et al. 1993). So far, resistance arguments do not justify the adoption of any specific product or range of products or the use of different products in rotation or mosaic. The most pressing research need is to find nonpyrethroid insecticides suitable for ITNs. Even products that sterilize female mosquitoes rather than killing them could still be useful in mixures with pyrethroids (Curtis et al. 1993; Miller 1994b). Resistance monitoring is important whenever insecticides are used on a large scale. Magesa et al. (1994) have assessed methods that use the World Health Organization (WHO) susceptibility-testing kit to detect pyrethroid resistance in *Anopheles* mosquitoes .

After a treatment session, people should be asked for reports of insecticidal activity; absence of effect against mosquitoes or other nuisance insects might be the first sign of resistance. It could also indicate that the treatment was not done correctly — equally valuable information. However, user's reports should not be regarded as an adequate substitute for essential monitoring of resistance and operational quality control.

Effects on nuisance arthropods

People use nets mostly to protect themselves from nuisance biting; protection from disease is secondary (Zandu et al. 1991; Aikins et al. 1993; Stephens et al. 1995) (also see Chapter 4). ITNs seem less lethal to *Culex quinquefasciatus* mosquitoes than *Anopheles* species, although they are fairly effective at preventing *C. quinquefasciatus* from biting (Curtis et al. 1991; Magesa et al. 1991; Curtis et al. 1994). This property would be especially important in urban areas, where *C. quinquefasciatus* is responsible for most nuisance biting. Failure to reduce the perceived nuisance of mosquito biting would probably jeopardize any urban ITN program.

Seasonal changes in nuisance biting can affect ITN use. In Bagamoyo, Tanzania, for example, the proportion of people using ITNs declined at the beginning of the dry season, when mosquito density was low but sporozoite rates (and hence infection risk) remained high (J.N. Minjas, personal communications).

Users often appreciate the effect pyrethroid-impregnated nets have on other arthropod pests, such as bedbugs, chicken ticks, headlice, and cockroaches (Charlwood and Dagoro 1989; Lindsay, Snow, Armstrong et al. 1989) as much as they do the effect on mosquitoes (Njunwa et al. 1991).

Nets, Curtains, and Other Fabrics

Net design

Both conical and rectangular nets are common in many places. Conical nets are easier to hang and fold up. Ease of use is particularly important in small rooms where the beds are used as seats or tables during the day. Rectangular nets, on the other hand, can hang from string as well as from frames and are more spacious inside. This presumably reduces the chance of lying against the netting, especially when there are several occupants.

More important for net treatment is whether the bottom border or top of the net is made of heavier, more absorbent material. A sheeting border prevents snagging and tearing when the net is tucked under the mattress, and at the top of a conical net, sheeting reinforces the weight-bearing apex. Unfortunately, sheeting tends to absorb much more liquid than netting, especially if the sheeting is cotton and the netting synthetic. When a reinforced net is dipped, therefore, a large and usually unknown fraction of the insecticide is taken up by sheeting tops and borders, where it is presumably much less effective. Testing of ITNs in Dar es Salaam, Tanzania, suggests that, on average, more than half the insecticide used to treat them was wasted in this way (J.E. Miller and J. Lines, unpublished). Therefore, it is also more difficult to calculate the dilution needed to achieve a specific dosage of insecticide on the netting.

These problems can be minimized by making nets with detachable borders and tops or by making narrow borders of relatively nonabsorbent synthetic fabric. These problems can be avoided altogether by giving up the advantages of dipping and spraying the net instead. Another potential solution, which seems as yet untried, is binding the border with plastic and string, as in tie-dyeing. Net designs and preference issues are discussed further in Chapter 3.

Netting material

The fabrics most commonly used for ITNs are cotton, cotton–synthetic blends, nylon, polyester, polyethylene, and polypropylene. These materials vary widely in their capacity to absorb dilute insecticide emulsion. It is not difficult to achieve a specific dosage if the amount of liquid the net will take is known; the insecticide can be diluted accordingly. However, it is a problem when different fabrics must be dipped together.

Cotton absorbs more emulsion than do synthetics. With permethrin, this difference may not matter: permethrin is less insecticidal on
cotton than on synthetic fibre (Miller 1994a; Elissa and Curtis 1995).
Therefore, the same dilution can be used for both cotton and nylon nets
because, although the cotton will absorb more permethrin, it needs more
to achieve the same effect. In Tanzania, a final dilution of about 1.0%
permethrin proved suitable. A similar difference between cotton and
nylon or polyester has also been seen with lambdacyhalothrin and
alphamethrin but not with deltamethrin (Figure 6) (Luo et al. 1994; Miller
1994a; Elissa and Curtis 1995).

The interaction between insecticide and fabric is complex and difficult to predict. Bioassays and experimental-hut studies have only begun
to explore combinations of fabric, compound, and dosage. Other aspects,
such as weight and type of weave, await consideration. Moreover, comparisons of the insecticidal power of freshly treated fabrics may be

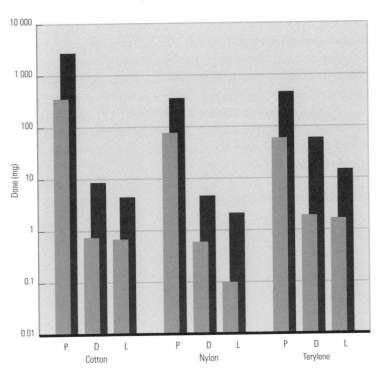

Figure 6. Estimates of LC$_{50}$ (■) and LC$_{90}$ (■) from 3-minute bioassays with *Anopheles gambiae* on netting
treated with a range of doses of permethrin (P), deltamethrin (D), and lambdacyhalothrin (L) (LC$_{50}$ and LC$_{90}$
are the concentrations lethal to 50 and 90%, respectively, of organisms tested) (source: Miller 1994a).

misleading. For example, immediately after treatment, a given concentration of insecticide is as active on polyethylene as it is on nylon or polyester, but on polyethylene this activity fades more rapidly with time and with washing (Curtis et al. 1994). Anecdotal evidence suggests that deltamethrin on polyethylene or polypropylene has more severe side effects than on other materials (C.F. Curtis, personal communication). Clearly, more information is needed, and research must accelerate if we are to keep up with new compounds and formulations.

The dipping process is also influenced by how thoroughly a fabric can be wrung. Light, flexible polyester and nylon nets can be wrung thoroughly after dipping so that very little emulsion drips out as the ITN dries. Cotton tends to drip even after thorough wringing and loses more insecticide. Polyethylene and polypropylene nets tend to be made of thick, rather stiff fibres and are difficult to wring at all. To save insecticide, freshly dipped ITNs can be allowed to drip onto plastic sheeting from which excess insecticide is collected for reuse (S.R. Meek, personal communication). Most of the excess drips out of a polyester ITN in a few minutes, but it can take much longer with a cotton one.

Durability is one of the most important determinants of the cost of nets, and a strong net is a more attractive purchase than a fragile one. Durability is measured in "denier," a scale of load-bearing strength; a 40-denier net is too flimsy, whereas 100-denier nets cost little more and are much sturdier. Stronger, more expensive nets are cheaper in the long run (in terms of dollars per year of effective life). This is discussed further in Chapter 3.

Fibre with incorporated insecticide

Techniques for improving the wash resistance of insecticide treatment have kindled some interest. Lindsay, Hossain et al. (1991) showed that a hot-acid treatment, which can be carried out at the factory, increased insecticide uptake and improved wash resistance. Techniques to incorporate the insecticide in the net fibre as it is produced are even more promising. Experimental-hut trials show that the initial insecticidal activity of Olyset™, a ready-made ITN manufactured by Sumitomo Corp., is similar to that of an ITN treated conventionally with the same dosage. The manufacturer's claims for greatly improved wash and wear resistance are currently being evaluated, and the early results are encouraging (C.F. Curtis, personal communication).

Unconventional bednets

An untreated net needs to be impenetrable to mosquitoes, but even nets with very wide mesh protect well after pyrethroid treatment. In Tanzania, ribbons of polypropylene made by stripping the warp from the weft of fertilizer sacks are used for treated bed curtains. Very incomplete as a physical barrier, these treated bed curtains protect well against biting, though not as well as treated nets (Curtis et al. 1994)

Nets versus curtains

Impregnated curtains over eaves, windows, and doors protect everyone in the room and may therefore be valuable in the evening before bedtime. In some places, such as Burkina Faso, they are a more practical alternative to nets because houses are very small or otherwise unsuitable for individual bednets (Pietra et al. 1991; Procacci et al. 1991). However, trials with pyrethroid-treated curtains show that they protect less well than similarly treated nets (Lines et al. 1987; Curtis et al. 1992; Beach et al. 1993). Recently, more encouraging results were achieved with curtains treated with the carbamate bendiocarb (Curtis et al. 1994).

The perfect ITN material for curtaining doors and windows has yet to be found. Conventional 100-denier netting proved unsuitable in Burkina Faso, where it tended to lose its shape and curl after 1 year of use. Investigators also reported that rodents eat eaves curtains (A. Habluetzel, personal communication).

Pyrethroid-treated wall curtains have been tried in Kenya. Called Mbu cloth, these consist of 9 m of sheeting affixed to the walls rather than the eaves or windows. Village-scale trials have been entomologically and epidemiologically inconclusive (Mutinga et al. 1992; Mutinga et al. 1993).

Insecticides

Synthetic pyrethroids were originally developed to mimic the insecticidal compounds in pyrethrum because natural pyrethrum is too unstable to use as a residual insecticide. Synthetic pyrethroids have several advantages for ITN use: they have excito-repellent properties and are quick acting and effective in the small quantities that will adhere to fabric.

Safety

In considering the safety of synthetic chemicals, three main kinds of short- and long-term hazard can be distinguished: to people, to nontarget organisms, and to the environment. Synthetic chemicals can present short- or long-term hazards to both humans and other nontarget organisms and to the environment. Anyone involved in ITN treatment and distribution should read the *Environmental Health Criteria* (EHC) booklets published by WHO (1990a,b,c), which discuss these risks. WHO's guardedly optimistic approach to pyrethroids contrasts strongly with its alarming statements about organophosphate and carbamate insecticides (WHO 1986a,b). Some of the more significant remarks about permethrin are reproduced in Table 3. The other booklets contain similar comments about lambdacyhalothrin and deltamethrin.

Pyrethroids have no tendency for bioaccumulation — in contrast to DDT, for example — and break down rapidly both in mammalian tissues and in the soil. Their toxicity for fish and other aquatic organisms, however, has important consequences for waste disposal. Pit latrines, in which pyrethroids degrade quickly, are recommended for this purpose.

For people, the rapid breakdown in tissue means that the main hazards of pyrethroids are related to acute rather than chronic exposure. For example, if all the insecticide on an ITN were absorbed completely

Table 3. Selected quotes on the safety of permethrin.

Environmental fate
- ❖ Permethrin degrades in soil, with a half-life of 28 days or less
- ❖ In general the degradative processes ... lead to less toxic products

Effects on nontarget organisms
- ❖ Permethrin is very toxic to fish and aquatic arthropods
- ❖ Permethrin is highly toxic to honey bees, but has very low toxicity to birds

Effects on experimental animals and *in vitro* test systems
- ❖ Permethrin is rapidly metabolised in tissue
- ❖ Permethrin has a low acute toxicity to rats, mice, rabbits and guinea pigs, though the LD_{50} value varies considerably according to the vehicle used and the *cis–trans* isomeric ratio
- ❖ There is no evidence for mutagenicity or teratogenicity
- ❖ There is no evidence for sensitization (allergic reactions)

Effects on human beings
- ❖ No fatal poisoning cases have ever been reported
- ❖ The likelihood of oncogenic effects in human beings is extremely low or nonexistent
- ❖ There are no indications that permethrin has adverse effects on humans when used as recommended

Source: WHO (1990a).

through a person's skin over 6 months, the amount absorbed would approach the estimated acceptable daily intake, which is 0.05 mg/kg for permethrin and a little less for deltamethrin and lambdacyhalothrin (Plestina 1989).

Insecticide hazards vary by formulation and mode of exposure. Formulation is important because the solvent itself may be harmful (see "Formulations," pp. 37–38). On contact with skin, some pyrethroids produce characteristic sensations (see "Side Effects," pp. 36–37).

We must also consider oral toxicity because insecticide packaged and sold for home ITN treatment could be swallowed by a child. Table 4 compares the amounts that might be sold in this way, using current standard doses, with LD_{50} values quoted in EHC booklets. The contents of a single sachet of an EC (emulsifiable concentrate) formulation comes uncomfortably close to the LD_{50} for rats. (LD_{50} is the amount required in a single dose to kill 50%, on average, of a group of test animals.) Although data on rats cannot be extrapolated reliably to humans and the insecticide usually has a strongly emetic effect, the figures suggest that a 10-kg child (about 1 year old) who swallowed an entire sachet could be seriously poisoned.

Table 4. Comparison between LD_{50} estimates (in rats) for three pyrethroids and the amount of insecticide needed to treat a single large bednet.

Compound	Rat LD_{50} (mg/kg)[a]		Maximum amount (mg) on one net
	Oral	Dermal	
Permethrin			
Technical			8 000[b]
In corn oil	500–5 000	>4 000	
Deltamethrin			
Technical		700	400[c]
In sesame oil	128		
2.5% EC	535		
2.5% flowable	22 000		
Lambdacyhalothrin			
Technical			400[c]
In corn oil	56	632	
10% CS	>5 000		

Source: WHO (1990a,b,c).
[a] LD_{50} is the dose that is lethal to 50% of animals tested.
[b] 500 mg/m², 16-m² bednet.
[c] 25 mg/m², 16-m² bednet.

This risk seems to be the gravest of those attached to a commercial market in net treatment. By contrast, the LD_{50} of each of the two water-based formulations (lambdacyhalothrin CS (microencapsulated) and deltamethrin flowable) is much greater, and the risk of serious poisoning, therefore, seems extremely remote.

These warnings are offset by the fact that permethrin and deltamethrin have been in agricultural use for many years (deltamethrin was first marketed in 1977). In that time, they have acquired an excellent reputation for safety.

He et al. (1989) reviewed 573 cases of acute pyrethroid poisoning in the Chinese medical literature. There were seven deaths, of which five were attributable directly to the pyrethroid rather than to any other chemical exposure or subsequent treatment. The vast majority of patients recovered within 6 days, and no residual symptoms were found. These cases mostly arose from occupational or accidental exposure to agricultural formulations, typically over a period of several days, and included some cases of attempted suicide. On the basis of the descriptions of four "illustrative cases," comparable degrees of occupational exposure could perhaps be anticipated in people who dip nets for a living, all day and every day, but would not normally be expected among people who are exposed occasionally to limited doses as they dip their own nets at home. Further discussion, specifically related to the use of cyfluthrin on nets, can be found in Bomann (1996).

Pyrethroids are already widely used in homes. For example, aerosol insecticides often contain a mixture of residual and nonresidual pyrethroids, typically amounting to 2.5 g in a large can. Permethrin is also used in lotions and shampoos for treating scabies and lice. Alpha-cyano compounds are considered less suitable for this purpose (Taplin and Meiking 1990). In 1995, the Food and Agriculture Organization of the United Nations was preparing guideline specifications for domestic pesticides for publication. The WHO (1991) comments on the requirements for registering pesticides for domestic use are reproduced in Box 6.

WHO frequently reiterates its approval of pyrethroids in general and of permethrin in particular for ITN treatment (WHO 1991). To date, however, WHO has not commented on safe insecticide-treatment practices. It should be asked to do so, particularly with respect to commercial products for home ITN treatment.

Box 6

Extract from *Safe Use of Pesticides* concerning household pesticides

The following general provisions should be considered before a pesticide is registered for household use:

1. Packaging should be firm, reclosable and so designed that the pesticide can be applied directly from the package. When a package is in a form in which a child might be able to get at its contents, its size should be such that the child could consume the whole contents without adverse effects.

2. The label should state what the product is and the pests against which it is effective, and give clear directions for use. All the information should be in local languages or dialects. The label should not be misleading and should not state that the contents are harmless to humans.

3. The date of manufacture should always be printed on the label. Registration authorities may require an expiry date, appropriate to local storage conditions, to be added.

4. The label should carry a specific and prominent warning against transfer of the contents to another container.

5. Any precautions that are needed, including where applicable the prevention of contamination of food, should be easy to carry out and very simply expressed.

6. Disposal of used containers, even with considerable residues of pesticide, should not require special precautions, so that they can be taken away with normal domestic refuse.

7. A person handling a household pesticide should not need to wear any type of special protective clothing.

8. The flammability, explosive potential and corrosiveness of solvents used in household pesticide formulations might present a greater hazard than the toxicity of the pesticide itself. The precautions needed to prevent the product catching fire or exploding should therefore be clearly indicated on the label.

Source: WHO (1991).

Side effects

Some solvents used in insecticide formulations have unpleasant effects. People who inhale solvent vapour for prolonged periods during dipping operations often suffer nonspecific, transient symptoms of mild intoxication, such as headaches. These effects can be avoided by dipping nets outdoors and by mixing the insecticide in a shallow basin rather than a deep bucket (Snow, Phillips et al. 1988).

Field reports of side effects from insecticide must distinguish permethrin from lambdacyhalothrin and deltamethrin. Permethrin has given rise to remarkably few reports of adverse side effects among ITN users or people involved in dipping. For example, Snow et al. (1987) asked the users of ITNs treated with permethrin or a placebo about nine different side effects, including headache, dizziness, coughing, sore eyes, and itching. The two groups differed only in that the placebo group complained more of sweating. In addition, one or two reports have referred to apparent allergic reactions, such as asthma and dermal sensitivity, on exposure during dipping (C. Reed and C.G. Nevill, personal communication). Such reactions seem remarkably rare, however.

Exposure of pyrethroids to skin, especially mucous membranes, can cause transient tingling and burning sensations known as paraesthesia. These symptoms are caused by temporary effects on sensory nerves, and no long-term adverse effects have been reported (WHO 1990b,c). Toxicologically, paraesthesia is regarded as having little significance beyond immediate discomfort; indeed, it is useful because it warns of exposure (WHO 1990c). Reports of paraesthesia from ITN treatment projects using permethrin are extremely rare, but it is commonly reported by people using alpha-cyano pyrethroids such as deltamethrin and lambdacyhalothrin (for example, Njunwa et al. 1991).

Two other effects have been reported with these compounds. First, the emulsion causes a painful irritation if splashed into the eye, and droplets of the concentrate produce a tingling sensation on contact with skin (Somboon 1993). Facial swelling has also been reported (Njunwa et al. 1991), possibly in connection with handling freshly dipped and dried ITNs, rather than with dipping itself. Second, people sleeping under freshly treated ITNs frequently report nasal irritation and sneezing lasting from a few days to 2 weeks after the ITN is first used.

These side effects have several operational consequences. In one trial in northwest Thailand, villagers cited such symptoms as one reason for washing their nets soon after treatment with lambdacyhalothrin

(Somboon 1993). In China, where deltamethrin is routinely used on millions of nets, such symptoms are rarely reported. In Tanzania, villagers sleeping under lambdacyhalothrin-treated nets noted nasal irritation (Njunwa et al. 1991) but stressed that they preferred it to the mosquitoes. Finally, in India, villagers reported skin tingling as a positive sign of the presence and strength of the deltamethrin used to treat their nets (Jana-Kara et al. 1995).

Severe or fatal illness soon after the introduction of ITNs is rarely reported. These stories are usually anecdotal and difficult or impossible to investigate properly. Before they come to official attention, they circulate as rumours, causing anxiety that hinders treatment operations (W. Fischer and Z. Premji, personal communication). It is unlikely that exposure to the insecticide deposit on an ITN could cause severe illness, and it must, therefore, be stressed that the insecticide was almost certainly not to blame in such cases. Our assertions of safety, however, can hardly be confident and convincing if we ignore exceptional cases. Little information on the side effects of ITNs exists, and a clearing house for this kind of information is urgently needed.

Formulations

Emulsifiable concentrates (ECs) are the pyrethroid formulations most commonly used for ITNs. They are easy to recognize because they are clear, often yellowish, liquid concentrates that turn milky when mixed with water. ECs contain solvents that are important not only because they can be toxic but also because they help the pyrethroid penetrate the skin. For this reason, formulations with a high insecticide content and less solvent per unit of volume, such as permethrin 55 %, should not necessarily be regarded as more toxic than formulations with less insecticide and more solvent. The solvent often gives freshly treated ITNs a characteristic odour (the insecticide itself is odourless), and although this odour disappears rapidly when the ITN is used, it can influence acceptability and perceptions of safety (Evans 1994).

Many manufacturers make different EC formulations for public-health and for agricultural use. Sometimes, the only important difference is the label, but sometimes the agricultural product contains more hazardous solvents. The national program in The Gambia rejected a whole batch of agricultural permethrin because it was not suitable for ITNs (M.K. Cham, personal communication). It is, therefore, important to order ECs formulated specifically for public-health applications.

Wettable powder (WP) formulations, normally used for spraying hard surfaces, are not generally suitable for ITNs. ITNs treated with permethrin WP lose their insecticidal effect within a few weeks (Miller 1990), probably because the powder simply falls off. Deltamethrin, on the other hand, seems about as effective in WP formulations as in EC formulations (Jana-Kara et al. 1994; Elissa and Curtis 1995; Jana-Kara et al. 1995).

Some formulations have solvents and insecticide suspended as an emulsion in water (for example the microencapsulated (CS) and the emulsion oil-in-water (EW)). These reduce skin absorbency somewhat and oral toxicity significantly (see Table 4), making them preferable for domestic use. Water-based formulations are available, in one form or another, for most pyrethroids used on ITNs — although, unfortunately, not for permethrin. Water-based formulations seem as effective for ITNs as equivalent ECs (for example, Elissa and Curtis 1995), but it is not yet clear whether they help to reduce paraesthesia.

One clear need is a formulation that is easy to use in small quantities — for example, a solid, divisible block that dissolves or disperses in water. Washing is a major influence on the residual effect of an insecticide deposit, and a "wash-proof" permethrin formulation has been investigated. So far, only marginal improvements have been achieved (Miller 1994a; Miller et al. 1995).

Choosing the right insecticides

Permethrin

Permethrin, one of the first synthetic pyrethroids with stable residual activity (WHO 1990a), was the first pyrethroid specifically recommended by WHO for ITN use. Permethrin is normally used at 200–500 mg/m^2 on nets, although higher doses have been used on curtains. At 200–500 mg/m^2, bioassays and experimental-hut studies indicate that re-treatment is required every 6 months if the net is not washed (Curtis et al. 1994). Washing removes about half the permethrin and rather more than half of the insecticidal activity (Hossain and Curtis 1989; Lindsay, Adiamah et al. 1991) (the consequences of this are discussed in "Packing, Dosage, and Re-treatment," pp. 42–45).

Little is known of other external factors determining the residual activity of the insecticide deposit on an ITN. The deposit seems to be affected remarkably little by soot and dirt but is reduced by handling

(Curtis et al. 1991). Permethrin is more insecticidal on synthetic fabrics than on cotton (see "Netting Material," pp. 28–30).

Experimental-hut comparisons have repeatedly shown that with synthetic fabric, increasing the dose beyond 200 mg/m^2 does not significantly improve either immediate insecticidal activity or residual activity (see Figure 5) (Curtis et al. 1994). Also, higher doses cost more (see Chapter 3). However, given the variability in doses actually achieved in routine dipping operations (see "Target Doses and Observed Doses," in this chapter, pp. 50–52), a safety margin in the target dose is desirable. Permethrin exists as two isomers, *cis* and *trans*. The *cis* form is more insecticidal but also more toxic to mammals (WHO 1990a). Formulations are available containing *cis–trans* isomer ratios of either 40 : 60 or 25 : 75. One manufacturer's suggestion that the latter formulation is preferable for public-health purposes does not seem justified. WHO (1990a), made no distinction between the two isomer ratios in its acceptable daily intake recommendation, and no major performance differences have emerged from experimental-hut trials (see Figure 5) (Pleass et al. 1993). In any case, the difference in *cis* isomer content is marginal compared with the large variations in the amounts applied per net in routine operations (Alonso, Lindsay, Armstrong-Schellenberg, Konteh et al. 1993).

Deltamethrin, lambdacyhalothrin, and other alpha-cyano compounds

Deltamethrin and lambdacyhalothrin belong to the subgroup of pyrethroids characterized by an alpha-cyano group in the molecular structure (WHO 1990b,c,d). These compounds are more toxic to mammals than permethrin, but their much greater toxicity to insects compensates for this (WHO 1990b). Therefore, remarkably little is needed on an ITN: 10–25 mg/m^2. Perhaps because small quantities adhere better to the substrate, the residual activity of nets treated with deltamethrin and lambdacyhalothrin can persist for 1 year, even with one or two washings (Njunwa et al. 1991; Curtis et al. 1992; Miller 1994a). This is a major advantage, especially in places where the malaria-transmission season lasts for more than 6 months a year. Some alpha-cyano compounds are, like permethrin, more effective on synthetics than on cotton (see "Netting Material," pp. 28–30; also see Figure 6).

Alpha-cyano pyrethroids are cheaper per individual treatment than permethrin (see Chapter 3). Their main disadvantage is that, on contact with skin, they can cause sensory side effects (see "Side Effects," pp. 36–37).

Currently, therefore, the choice is between more expensive compounds that require re-treatment every 6 months but are generally free of noticeable side effects and cheaper ones that are not. It is difficult to predict which product customers would choose to buy in a shop.

Other alpha-cyano compounds, such as cyfluthrin and alphamethrin, have also been tested in experimental-hut and village trials (Luo et al. 1994; Curtis et al. 1996). These compounds are not reviewed here; although alphamethrin has been used remarkably cheaply in China (Luo et al. 1994), none of these other compounds has yet proved outstanding in comparison with products already in common use.

Etofenprox

Etofenprox is a novel compound structurally different from, but functionally similar to, conventional pyrethroids. The dosage is similar to, that of permethrin, and it performs like permethrin in experimental hut trials (C.F. Curtis, personal communication). Its main advantage is its remarkably low toxicity to mammals — much lower even than permethrin. Because its structure is different, it is reasonable to assume that mosquito populations that have evolved resistance to conventional pyrethroids would be susceptible to etofenprox; unfortunately, this has not proved true of permethrin-resistant *An. stephensi* (Curtis 1992d).

Nonpyrethroid insecticides

Not many conventional nonpyrethroids are safe enough for ITNs. Moreover, in experimental huts, nets impregnated with the organophosphate pyrimiphos-methyl did not give good protection against biting, although many mosquitoes were killed (Miller 1994a). The carbamate bendiocarb is probably too toxic for nets, but on curtains it can both protect against biting and kill mosquitoes that enter the room (Curtis et al. 1994). However, Munasinghe (1994) found that in Sri Lankan houses, curtains treated with permethrin or lambdacyhalothrin prevented mosquito bites better than curtains treated with bendiocarb.

Actors and Organizations

ITNs need regular re-treatment, and this is a major obstacle to making ITN technology widely available. The insecticide must be transported from the manufacturer to the user, perhaps being repackaged on the way, and must then be applied to the net or curtain. Two kinds of people are likely to take part in this process: business people — including importers, wholesalers, and retailers — and the staff of public-health and community development organizations (Figure 7).

The insecticide is most likely to be distributed in the following ways:

❖ *Pretreatment*: An initial treatment is applied at the factory, warehouse, or shop before the nets are transported, distributed, or sold.

❖ *Coordinated treatment*: The nets or curtains of a whole community are treated and re-treated all together in an operation organized and supervised by trained people.

❖ *Individual treatment*: Owners decide when their nets or curtains need re-treatment and bring them to a shop or health facility to be treated by trained staff.

❖ *Home treatment*: Owners treat their own nets and curtains at home with small quantities of insecticide packaged for domestic use.

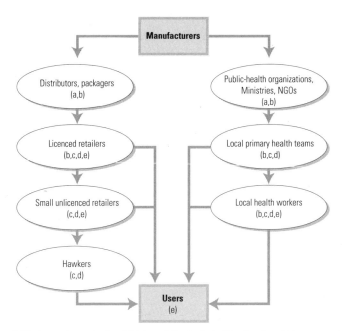

Figure 7. The two major routes by which insecticide for bednet treatment could be conveyed from manufacturer to user: (a) packaging, distributing, preparing information; (b) bulk impregnation of bednets; (c) selling and distributing treated bednets; (d) selling and distributing dip-it-yourself kits (sachets); (e) impregnating individual bednets.

Each method has advantages and disadvantages in training, logistics, and quality control. For example, pretreatment seems an efficient way to begin an ITN program, but it merely postpones the question of how re-treatment is to be organized and precludes the opportunity to demonstrate correct treatment methods from the start.

ITN programs are usually run by large- and medium-sized public-health organizations and are usually of the coordinated-treatment type. Outside the public-health context, pest-control companies may be able to develop a small market in mass ITN treatment for institutions such as schools and prisons.

Individual treatment, on the other hand, will probably be essential to the development of a viable domestic market in ITNs and will make public-health operations more flexible.

In some developed countries, home-treatment kits with small quantities of emulsifiable concentrate are already marketed for tourists. In developing countries, however, the domestic market remains uncertain, so relatively little effort has gone into adapting the technology so that it can be used for treatment services or for home use. Developing this market would make ITNs more available; the commercial and public-health distribution systems would complement each other, as they do with chloroquine.

National and international regulatory authorities are also important. They are responsible for ensuring that minimum safety standards are met throughout manufacture, distribution, and use of ITNs. This involvement includes approving the specifications of insecticide formulations and packaging and registering trade-marked products. It may also include a retail licencing system and inspections to check storage and handling practices, to prevent adulteration, and to ensure minimum standards of training. In some countries, existing regulations for pesticide distribution and use may be adequate, but no consensus exists on the specific criteria that should be applied in this case.

Processes

Packaging, dosage, and re-treatment

Most insecticides come in 0.5- to 2-L bottles or 20-L drums. These quantities are suitable for mass treatment; 1 L of 55% permethrin or 2.5% lambdacyhalothrin contains enough insecticide for 150 treatments (assuming doses of 200 and 10 mg/m^2, respectively, and 15 m^2 of fabric).

When insecticide is poured from 20-L drums, large amounts are spilled. Bottles are priced a little higher, but, as little is spilled, the true cost is probably about equal. Spillage also occurs during measuring, so squeeze-and-pour bottles are increasingly popular. These have two chambers: a reservoir in the bottom and a smaller, graduated chamber above. When the bottle is squeezed, the contents are forced from the reservoir into the graduated chamber, which can be emptied without releasing any more from the reservoir. These bottles are probably too big for home use, however. The domestic market will probably depend on individual treatments, especially in countries where even such items as mosquito coils and cigarettes are sold singly.

Individual doses of insecticide concentrate could be poured from a large bottle into smaller, reusable containers at point of sale. This method has two hazards, however: spillage and adulteration. Spillage could be minimized if insecticide were available in squeeze-and-pour bottles. Deliberate adulteration would be harder to control. Purchasers would not be able to detect dilution of a water-based formulation with water or of an EC with an organic solvent, such as kerosene. Reusable containers are, therefore, prohibited in some countries.

If insecticides are to be sold in small quantities, they must be packaged appropriately in sealed sachets or bottles with tamper-proof lids. Unfortunately, most formulations contain solvents that are incompatible with the plastics of which sachets and small bottles are usually made. This problem is not insurmountable: fluorinated or foil-laminated plastics can be used. AgrEvo already produces a foil sachet for Thailand (J. Invest, personal communication). However, factory-sealed sachets are expensive except in extremely large quantities. For example, one AgrEvo sachet containing 15 mL of permethrin worth less than $0.50 costs $1.60 each in quantities up to 20 000. With distribution costs and wholesalers' and retailers' markup, these sachets could not be sold for less than $2.50 — far too much for developing countries. This problem raises two questions: why not package insecticides for home use locally, and what are the technical standards for sachets to contain insecticides (Tincknell 1985; Dollimore 1993).

It is also difficult to specify the correct quantity and dilution for all combinations of insecticides and fabrics. As we have seen, the same dilution of permethrin suits both cotton and nylon, but the problem of quantity remains — cotton is more absorbent than nylon. Whatever quantity is chosen, it is probably too much for a small, light, synthetic net and not enough for large, heavy, cotton net. The AgrEvo 15-mL sachet is useful because it contains about 8 g of permethrin; diluted in 1 L of water, this quantity is enough for two medium-sized nylon nets treated at about 200 mg/m^2 or one fairly light cotton net treated at about 500 mg/m^2.

The aim with alpha-cyano compounds, on the other hand, is a consistent dosage, and cotton and synthetics require different dilutions to achieve this because they absorb different amounts of water. Ideally, therefore, users should choose between two different dilutions, depending on the fabric in their net. This could be made easier by supplying a plastic bag marked with two lines indicating the volumes of water for each type of fabric. It would be simpler, however, to specify a single intermediate dosage.

In fact, it is doubtful that dosages calculated for public-health programs are appropriate for home use. These doses are designed to maximize the treatment cycle and minimize the work load. Little is known about how often nets are normally washed, but several times over 6 months seems likely, especially where they are common. White nets are washed more often than coloured ones. Perhaps users could treat nets frequently with small doses during the last rinse of a monthly wash, as is often done with bleach or blueing. Such usage would also bring down the price of individual doses. According to one survey, this "little-and-often" expenditure pattern explains why urban Tanzanians spend more on mosquito coils than on nets (Stephens et al. 1995). It is not clear whether a little-and-often treatment system is feasible; an initial "loading dose" might be necessary.

Whatever the dosage, instructions are always a problem. This problem is partly a matter of conveying information clearly: it must be simple and in easily understood language. Pictures and pictograms should be used as much as possible, especially for safety warnings (Dollimore 1993). Measuring could be difficult; soft-drink or beer bottles could help — they come in standard sizes — but might users be tempted to put excess insecticide back in the bottle where an unsuspecting person might find it and drink it? Of course, users sometimes fail to follow even the clearest instructions, and everyone makes mistakes; for example, it is easy to lose count of the number of times one has filled a bottle and emptied it into a bucket. It is important to note, however, that unlike workers on a mass-treatment project, users dipping their own nets are probably not repeatedly and frequently exposed to insecticides, so greater latitude in procedure is acceptable.

Treatment techniques

Except in Central Africa, spraying is not common for ITN treatment outside China. It is, however, the routine treatment in Sichuan Province, where there are more pyrethroid ITNs than in all Africa (Curtis 1992b; Cheng et al. 1995). With spray pumps and skilled workers, spraying is quicker than dipping; also, it can be done without moving the net. However, it can be wasteful (Rozendaal et al. 1989; S.R. Meek, personal communication) and can produce patchier insecticide deposit. This latter effect does not seem to have been investigated.

Snow, Phillips et al. (1988), Curtis (1992c), and Sexton (1994) have all described ITN dipping techniques. Box 7 gives the essential details for nets made of a single fabric, and Figure 8 (A–D) shows the key steps in the treatment procedure.

Measuring absorptive capacity and area

Calculating the dilutions is clearly the most complicated aspect of net treatment. Achieving the right dose depends on a correct estimate of the net's area and the volume of water it will absorb. This volume can be measured by weighing the net first dry and then wet. Alternatively, the net can be soaked in a known volume of water, wrung out, and allowed to drip so that the excess water falls back into a bucket. The final volume of water in the bucket is measured, and the difference between this and the original volume is the amount of water retained by the net.

It would be helpful to have a rule for calculating absorptive capacity, but it is not easy to define. The volume absorbed per square metre depends not only on the material (synthetic or cotton), but also on whether the thread is monofilament or spun fibre, whether the fabric is woven or knit, and on the tightness of the mesh. The volume absorbed per kilogram of material may be less variable, as suggested by the data in Table 5. Recent work in Dar es Salaam suggests that 1g of fabric absorbs about 1mL of water, for a wide variety of nets (J.E. Miller, personal communication).

Where nets come in a range of standard sizes and materials, time and effort can be saved by drawing up a chart of appropriate volumes of water and insecticide for dipping different types, sizes, and numbers of nets.

As explained above, permethrin can be used in the same dilution to treat both cotton and synthetic nets. With deltamethrin, by contrast, the higher absorptive capacity of cotton must be compensated for with

Box 7

Net-dipping procedures

1. **Precautions**

   ❖ Dipping should be done in the open air or in a well-ventilated building.

   ❖ Long rubber gloves are desirable for short periods of work with alpha-cyano pyrethroids, such as deltamethrin or lambdacyhalothrin. They are essential for long periods of work with any insecticide.

   ❖ People dipping nets every day should wear protective clothing, such as coveralls and rubber boots.

   ❖ Avoid touching the face with hands contaminated with insecticide, especially alpha-cyano pyrethroids.

   ❖ Wash hands and clothing thoroughly when dipping is finished. Dump excess insecticide and empty packaging in a pit latrine or bury it.

2. **Materials**

   ❖ Bednets — wash immediately before treatment

   ❖ Insecticide:

   – Small measure, such as a 100-mL graduated cylinder

   – Large measure, such as a 1-L graduated cylinder

   – Mixing container, such as a plastic bag (suitable for one net), a plastic bowl, bucket, or bin (wide, shallow bowls are preferable to minimize concentration of solvent vapour)

   ❖ Water

3. **Measure water**

   ❖ Measure the water absorbed by a single net.

   ❖ Multiply this amount by the number of nets to be dipped and put that much water in the mixing container.

(continued)

Box 7 *(concluded)*

4. Measure insecticide

❖ Measure the area of one net in m^2.

❖ Multiply the area by the target dosage in mg/m^2; this gives the amount of pure insecticide required in milligrams (for example, $12\ m^2 \times 200\ mg/m^2 = 2\ 400\ mg$)

❖ Divide the result by the concentration of the insecticide in mg/mL (remember, 25% concentrate has 250 mg/mL), giving the volume of concentrate required by one net (for example, 2400 mg ÷ 250 mg/mL = 9.6 mL)

❖ Multiply this result by the number of nets to be dipped.

❖ Measure out that much concentrate, add it to the water in the mixing container, and mix.

5. Dip nets

❖ Before beginning treatment, ensure that nets are dry and clean.

❖ Soak each net completely for a few seconds.

❖ Wring the net thoroughly so that excess fluid drips into the dipping container.

❖ If necessary, especially with polyethylene nets, allow the net to drip over plastic sheeting for a few minutes.

6. Dry ITNs

❖ Lay ITNs flat on beds or on plastic sheeting or hang them up. Avoid exposing them to direct sunlight for more than a few hours. Ensure that they dry evenly.

❖ To ensure that they dry evenly, fold them as little as possible and turn them occasionally as they dry.

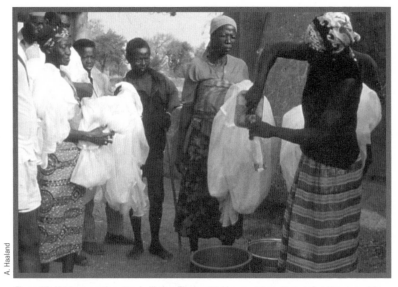

Figure 8A. Net impregnation, step 1: dilution. The insecticide concentrate is poured out into a container, allowing the volume to be measured carefully, and is then mixed with the water in a basin.

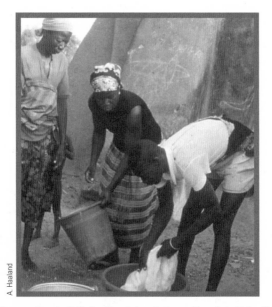

Figure 8B. Net impregnation, step 2: dipping. The whole net is thoroughly wetted with the diluted insecticide. Note that the people in this photo are not wearing gloves; they are householders treating their own nets. Rubber gloves should be used by workers who dip other people's nets and who, as a result, handle the insecticide repeatedly.

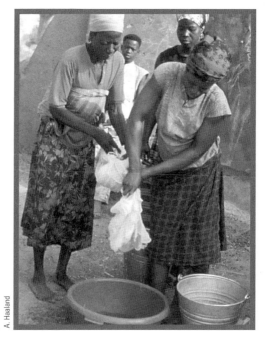

A. Haaland

Figure 8C. Net impregnation, step 3: wringing. The net is squeezed hard so that the excess liquid is returned to the bucket. If this is not done thoroughly, dilute insecticide will be wasted as it drips out of the drying net.

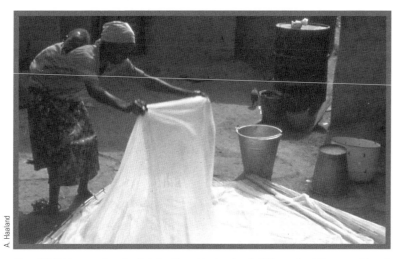

A. Haaland

Figure 8D. Net impregnation, step 4: drying. The net is placed so that it has as few folds as possible and is turned over occasionally as it dries.

Table 5. Absorbency in relation to area and weight of two types of bednets.

Origin	Type of material	Area (m^2)	Weight (g)	Volume absorbed (mL)
Mali	Cotton–polyamide sides; percale top and border	22	1 500	1 500
Thailand	Polyester, 100 denier	14.5	460	500

a more dilute emulsion; therefore, separate dilutions would be necessary for cotton and synthetic nets.

Target doses and observed doses

Netting absorbs insecticide in proportion to the volume of emulsion it takes up. In other words, insecticide is not differentially absorbed, and when many nets are dipped together, the first picks up neither more nor less insecticide than the last (Hossain et al. 1989).

In the laboratory, chemical assays usually indicate that actual dosages vary moderately but are, on average, fairly close to the target (Hossain et al. 1989; Lindsay, Adiamah et al. 1991; Miller et al. 1991). This finding is also sometimes the experience in the field (Snow, Phillips et al. 1988).

In other cases, however, surprising differences have been reported between the average amount of insecticide that should have been taken up during a mass dipping and the amount later found on netting samples (for example, Somboon 1993). In The Gambia, Alonso, Lindsay, Armstrong-Schellenberg, Konteh et al. (1993) calculated from the amount of insecticide used and the number of net treatments recorded that, on average, 1 183 mg had been consumed per square metre of netting, compared with a target dosage of 500 mg/m^2. Chemical assays on random samples taken shortly afterward from villages showed a mean dose of only 179 mg/m^2. This discrepancy may have been caused by insecticide dripping out of nets as they dried.

On the whole, relatively little attention has been paid to variations in the insecticide deposit from net to net or to patchiness of deposits. The field project by Alonso and co-workers is unusual because it produced such information. Deposits on individual ITNs were patchy; three samples were taken from each ITN, and the mean range across a net was 285 mg/m^2. Variation between nets was even greater (Figure 9), and surprisingly little of this variation could be attributed to differences among villages and net materials. Patchiness may or may not be functionally important, but variation from net to net certainly is. We need to know more about what causes it.

Some dipping methods have been adopted, retained, and communicated for reasons that make sense but have never been tested experimentally. For example, some groups recommend drying ITNs flat, whereas others hang them up. The method that gives a more even distribution of insecticide has not apparently been identified. Rozendaal et al. (1989) showed that ITNs hung to dry vertically have a slight downward gradient in insecticide concentration, although the difference between top and bottom was negligible compared with the variation observed by Alonso and co-workers in The Gambia. Preliminary experiments with ink dissolved in the concentrate suggest that orientation is

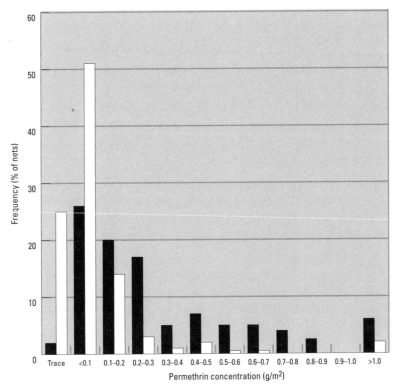

Figure 9. Frequency distribution of permethrin concentrations measured on routinely treated nets in The Gambia soon after impregnation (June, ■) and later in the season (November, ☐) (source: Alonso, Lindsay, Armstrong-Schellenberg, Konteh et al. 1993).

not as important as folding; colour accumulates at drying points, such as the edges of folds (J. Lines, unpublished).

Conclusions and Recommendations

In Africa, most scientific ITN trials have concentrated on entomological or epidemiological impact. Projects designed to establish practical methods for routine implementation have distributed large numbers of ITNs. The main outstanding problem is how to make re-treatment available in a sustainable manner that achieves consistently good coverage.

This review shows that technical, operational, and social questions are mutually dependent; the solution to an operational problem will usually raise technical questions, and vice versa. Wider implementation demands study of the following technical issues:

❖ Developing a simple way to quantify insecticide deposits on ITNs;

❖ Improving the repeatability and standardization of bioassays and field tests for monitoring mosquito resistance to pyrethroids;

❖ Investigating resistance — increasing the intensity of surveillance, verifying field reports, and studying biochemical mechanisms and ways to delay resistance evolution;

❖ Standardizing laboratory methods for comparing netting–insecticide combinations and expanding this work to new compounds and different field conditions;

❖ Comparing the ease and effectiveness of various net-treatment procedures, including spraying, taking into account the diversity of net designs and fabrics, and identifying sources of variation in the dosages produced in routine dipping; and

❖ Improving packaging — comparing the convenience and safety of various forms of packaging (and their attached instructions) for both public-health use and commercial sale and identifying public preferences with respect to packaging and dipping methods.

General recommendations for research include the following:

❖ Setting up an effective monitoring system for reports of pyrethroid toxicity during treatment and use of ITNs;

❖ Establishing an international consensus on regulating the commercial marketing of pyrethroids for ITNs, including choice of insecticide and formulation; setting standards for packaging, handling, and labeling; and licencing distributors and retailers;

❖ Continuing the search for pyrethroid and nonpyrethroid insecticides suitable for ITNs; and

❖ Developing a netting fibre incorporating a long-acting insecticide and other procedures to increase wash resistance and lengthen re-treatment intervals.

Chapter 3

Experiences of Implementation

R.M. Feilden

T his chapter reviews the operational experiences of schemes and programs using nets or curtains impregnated with insecticide as an intervention against malaria. The discussion applies almost equally to nets and curtains, so the phrase "insecticide-treated nets" (ITNs) is used throughout. The review covers ITN interventions conducted as primary health care (PHC) services, as well as more vertical or selective ITN interventions. The operational cases range from national programs to schemes for smaller populations, such as a hospital's clientele. Examples have been sought from the public sector, the private sector, international donors, and nongovernmental organizations (NGOs).

Most of the literature reflects the principal objective of field trials: demonstrating the efficacy of ITN technology. The details of planning, supervising, managing, and monitoring the implementation of an ITN program are not typically covered in scientific journals. The information used in this review appears mostly in training manuals, household surveys, recording and reporting formats, shipping documents, and annual reports. These sources describe delays, hurdles, and setbacks as well as achievements. I am indebted to everyone who answered our questions; however, the information we obtained does not constitute a complete review of implementation in practice.

This review takes an approach frequently used in external evaluations of health programs. It considers both inputs (such as supplies and staff) and the activities and processes that must take place if the inputs are to achieve the desired result. This approach does not attempt to evaluate outcomes, such as changes in morbidity and mortality. It mirrors the method for evaluating the Expanded Programme on Immunization (EPI), in which the quality of immunization services is assessed not by sero-conversion surveys or tests of vaccine potency, but by combining measures of utilization with indicators of cold-chain quality, staff technique for handling vaccine and administering injections, and stock management. The assumption is that inputs and activities of a defined and acceptable quality are needed to produce the desired outcome. In an ITN program, the objective is a properly impregnated net that is used correctly. Process evaluation permits identification and rectification of operational constraints. One objective of this review is to identify indicators that will help managers to implement, monitor, and evaluate ITN activities.

We obtained little information about private-sector inputs and activities, so this review concentrates on ITN programs implemented by governments, international donors, NGOs, and not-for-profit ventures. The effect of subsidized programs on private suppliers is of particular interest, as are administrative and legal constraints that businesses and NGOs face to a far greater extent than do international agencies.

Does the Supply of Bednets and Insecticide Meet Demand?

Is there any need for market intervention to make ITNs more readily available? Household surveys and ITN projects introduced by employers, NGOs, and donors suggest that ITNs would be used more widely if they were available and if people could afford to buy them.

Nets have been used for decades, but the market shows both uneven supply and lack of knowledge among potential customers. On the supply side, there are places, such as Maputo in Mozambique, where people know about nets and were in the habit of using them but now cannot find them in the shops. In other places, such as Dar es Salaam (Evans 1994) and Bobo-Dioulasso (Guiguemde et al. 1994), both urban wage-earning communities, nets are sold but many people do not have the money to buy them at open-market prices. In a third category, people would like nets but local traders do not stock them (perhaps because of insufficient demand at the open-market price); however, the local project can make nets at much lower cost than the price charged at the nearest supply outlet. This situation has been reported from Turkana in northern Kenya (J. Miesen, personal communication). In some places, houses are too small for nets, so other insecticide-treated textile barriers, such as curtains, are more appropriate. Elsewhere, people are compelled by their occupation or lifestyle to be outdoors and exposed to mosquitoes during peak biting time, as reported from Bagamoyo, Tanzania (Makemba et al. 1995), and Vietnam (Marchand 1994). This mixed profile of market conditions indicates that strategies must be tailored to each situation.

Although a public-health service may work to get as many people as possible to sleep under nets, flooding the market with subsidized nets will not necessarily produce the intended result. An influx of low-cost nets may challenge traders to lower their prices, but this action might rapidly undermine the private sector, which faces import duties, delays, and losses from which international donors are insulated by their status. Both donors and governments should, therefore, review the local net market carefully before launching large-scale programs. The Program for Appropriate Technology in Health (PATH) is currently conducting such a review in several African countries (PATH 1995).

Providing nets below market price offers an opportunity for windfall gains to people who choose to resell their subsidized nets. This experience is also a common feature of subsidized housing schemes: some families prefer to lease or sell their new house because its market value exceeds their perception of the benefit of improved accommodation. Therefore, nets must be offered at prices that are sustainable for both sellers and buyers. The puzzle is how to make the nets available without destroying the private sector, which users must rely on when donor funding ends. Equity must also enter the equation: ITN interventions should include subsidies for people who cannot afford even the "sustainable" price.

Compared with the market for nets, the market for public-health insecticides is in its infancy. Even in places where most people have been able to buy nets, ITNs are virtually unknown except through research projects, donor funding, or national programs. For example, in a sample of urban households in Dar es Salaam, 62% owned at least one net, 48% claimed to have heard of soaking nets in insecticide, but only 5% had an ITN, mostly acquired from projects such as the Urban Malaria Control Project (UMCP). Others had experimented with available chemicals. People who had heard of treatment learned about it from the donor-funded activities of the UMCP and rural ITN projects, newspapers, and the radio, not from the private sector (Evans 1994). The product is not yet available, or established as a complementary purchase, or recognized (indicated by people experimenting with available chemicals), which suggests that there is scope for marketing.

A study of household expenditure on malaria treatment and prevention in the town of Bobo-Dioulasso, Burkina Faso, found that 35% of the families surveyed used at least one net (Guiguemde et al. 1994). Impregnation was reported to be offered by the town health services at $0.10. The net-dipping service has been expanded (V. Curtis, personal communication).

The market for public-health insecticides is virtually nonexistent and is likely to remain under tight control. Few manufacturers make public-health-grade pyrethroids. Local regulations on the sale of pyrethroids constrain their availability. National control authorities responsible for licencing medical and public-health products must be convinced that products are safe and efficacious before permitting their import and sale. This problem was cited by a nonprofit organization selling ITNs in Zimbabwe (T. Freeman, personal communication). Taxes also constrain availability by raising import costs. In Tanzania, this constraint was removed when pyrethroids were classified as public-health products rather than as agricultural products. The extent to which the World Health Organization (WHO), donors, NGOs, and researchers should promote registration of suitable insecticides remains an open question.

Choosing a Macro-Level Strategy

Sources of finance and responsibility for logistics

ITN strategies can be characterized by

- ❖ Sources of finance; and
- ❖ Responsibility for distributing nets and offering treatment services.

For both financing and provision of supplies, there is a spectrum ranging from governments to households and including donors, NGOs, nonprofit organizations, employers, and businesses. Strategies are complicated by the fact that an ITN comprises two distinct products that may be financed and supplied from different sources. Table 6 shows how selected interventions fit into this matrix. Donors working through government health services have been counted as public sector, as have field trials requiring no financial contribution from ITN users.

Table 6. Matrix for sources of financing and responsibility for logistics.

Financing	Distribution, logistics, sales, and services		
	Public	Mixed	Private
Public	China (dipping and spraying) Ecuador (dipping) The Gambia (free dipping before 1993) Most field trials		
Mixed	Kenya (Bamako Initiative projects)	The Gambia (paid dipping after 1992) Tanzania (Bagamoyo project) NGO schemes such as in Afghanistan	Central African Republic (social marketing)
Private			China (nets) Ecuador (nets) The Gambia (nets) Employers

No examples were found of private financing combined with public distribution or of public financing combined with private distribution. The largest population of ITN users is in China, where users buy nets from the private sector, and the public sector supplies the insecticide. However, China's private sector is not strictly comparable with that in Africa or South America.

Supplying ITNs through the private sector

The private sector could be left to develop at its own pace or encouraged through financial incentives, such as reduced import duties or taxes. Either possibility raises questions about whether and how to monitor and regulate the advertising of insecticides and their quality, safety of use, and disposal. Public-information services might be needed to explain the merits of ITNs and to tell people how to use insecticide correctly. A comparison of mosquito-control measures used by households in Dar es Salaam suggests that ITNs would cost a family less than the current combinations of untreated nets, coils, and aerosol sprays (Evans 1994). If the private sector offers net-treatment services, customers must know how they can tell whether their net has been correctly treated (see also Chapters 2 and 4).

Employers' schemes, such as those launched at tea plantations in Malawi and Zimbabwe, are considered private-sector interventions. Such projects are introduced on the employer's initiative and funded partly from employees' wages.

In a social-marketing approach, the private sector becomes the main supplier of both nets and insecticide. The public sector (or NGOs and donors) might subsidize this type of project and promote the intervention (see also Chapter 4).

Supplying ITNs through a vertical strategy

Some public-sector interventions address malaria control as a vertical or selective activity. The UMCP in Dar es Salaam, which is supported by the Japan International Cooperation Agency (JICA), uses this approach, in which spraying teams have adopted ITNs as an additional method of vector control. In China, insecticide is provided as part of official vector-control activities and users supply their own nets. Ecuador and other South American countries may also use this model (Kroeger et al. 1995).

This approach depends on continued financial commitment from either the government or an external donor, but the long-term consequences of this dependence must be assessed.

Supplying ITNs through a strategy integrated with health services

In an integrated approach by the public sector, malaria prevention, treatment, and control are integrated with PHC services or district hospital services. This approach was chosen by the Kenyan government, with support from the United Nations Children's Fund (UNICEF). Malaria-control activities are part of the district-based Bamako Initiative projects and involve health workers from the community (including traditional birth attendants), the village health committee, the community pharmacy (through which nets are sold), and professional health staff at facility and district levels (for monitoring and supervision). Such an approach carries the risk of overloading community health workers with an ever-increasing number of activities, so this risk should be carefully considered. An integrated public-sector approach could deliver ITNs to high-risk groups — pregnant women and newborns — through mother and child health programs, including the EPI. Various levels of subsidy could be applied. To date, this approach has not been tried.

Can a macro-level strategy ensure equity of access to ITNs?

A major shortcoming of any approach that relies on the private sector is that access depends on disposable income; thus, equity is not assured. Under the vertical and the integrated strategies, mechanisms can be set up so that health services or the community, or both, can identify those who are without the protection of an ITN. The capacity to direct subsidized nets toward the most needy will probably be greatest in an integrated approach in rural areas.

In China's malarious provinces, private net ownership has been promoted through the public sector, which also provides the insecticide. In 1988, 3.85 million people in 42 counties in Sichuan Province were protected by nets; this represents 96.7% coverage (2.34 million nets, owned at a rate of 2.61 per household and occupied by 1.65 people per net) (Curtis 1992b). However, the socioeconomic factors that make this strategy feasible for China are not found in Africa.

In the absence of other strategies, some sections of the population will not be able to buy ITNs from the private sector. Even in the urban wage-earning economy of Dar es Salaam, 27% of respondents said they did not own a net because they could not afford the initial investment (Evans 1994). This problem is even more serious in rural areas such as Turkana, Kenya, where net ownership was constrained not only by lack of cash but also by the absence of nets in the local shops (J. Miesen, personal communication). The poorest, who can least afford to miss work because of illness, would be most at risk through lack of effective protection. So far, no evaluations of ITN interventions in Africa have been found that quantify how far the objective of equity has been achieved.

Have explicit policy choices been made?

The process of testing ITNs and then, on the basis of field trials, deciding to introduce national or regional ITN programs has been followed in China, The Gambia, Papua New Guinea, and the Solomon Islands. In Ecuador, scaling-up of field trials to national level is in process. Apart from technical evaluation of the coverage and quality of national ITN programs, policy research is needed to identify what must be done to scale up an intervention from a demonstration phase and to define the optimum combination of private- and public-sector efforts in a particular country. This research should consider not only socioeconomic characteristics, differences between urban and rural areas, and issues of logistics, such as travel costs and seasons when routes are impassable, but also the legal and administrative requirements for supporting a national ITN policy.

Choosing a Micro-Level Strategy

The details of ITN projects and programs depend on the existing situation. Do people already use nets? If yes, what are they made of and how big are they? If not, would they use them, given the chance? What type of net — shape, colour, size, and fabric — should be chosen?

Planning for ITN activities differs fundamentally from planning for other PHC activities in two ways: with ITNs, the client must provide the major item of equipment; and the dose is not determined at the point of manufacture, as with pills, or by skilled health staff, as with injections and drops. These factors are relevant whether users obtain ITNs from the public sector or from private sources. Clients' involvement in purchasing, maintaining, and using ITNs correctly introduces operational complications that make situation analysis an indispensable part of identifying appropriate and feasible strategies.

What information should be obtained in advance?

The starting point for a public-sector or NGO intervention is usually morbidity or mortality statistics indicating that malaria is a major health problem. Before launching an ITN scheme, the planners must gather information from both the health services and the intended clients. Developing the details of a strategy is an interactive process dependent on the capacity of health services and the response of the community. Strategies should be adjusted as experience accumulates.

Community-based schemes may arise from community interest or facilitators' suggestions. The process of developing a small intervention (for example, in a few villages or based on one hospital) can be far more organic and responsive than is possible at district or national levels. If the intervention is part of a holistic health and welfare improvement (for example, one including water-supply or income-generating activities), the operational procedures may depend on supporting factors that may not be present elsewhere. The many innovative ideas found in such schemes must be assessed on two criteria before assuming that they will apply on a wider basis: the size and density of the population covered and the ratio of outside managerial support personnel to the size of population.

Experience from field trials seldom gives much help with developing an operational strategy. The objective of these trials is to test impact on disease, not to develop sustainable structures for procuring and distributing equipment and supplies; getting the right dose of insecticide onto nets; monitoring record keeping, reporting, and financial management. Notable exceptions are the Bagamoyo project, which has a specific community component (Winch et al. 1993), and the trials in Ecuador and Peru (Kroeger et al. 1995), which are currently being scaled up for implementation by ministry of health staff.

The data to collect in preliminary surveys before introducing ITNs are set out in a WHO publication (WHO–VBC 1989). Several programs and trials have included a survey of baseline knowledge, attitudes, and practices. A review of the results emphasizes the importance of direct observation, checking the validity of responses, using open-ended questions rather than precoded answer categories, and avoiding leading questions ("When did you last have malaria?") and hypothetical questions ("How much would you be willing to pay?").

For example, in Yaoundé, Cameroon, two styles of questioning were used to investigate the nuisance caused by mosquitoes. In 1988, leading questions and precoded response categories were used, but in 1990 the questions were open ended (Louis et al. 1990). The surveys received similar answers for "mosquito bites" and "unpleasant noise" (53% and 21% versus 56% and 28%) and different results for "illness" (23% versus 3%). When asked an open-ended question, people seem more concerned with specific aspects of the nuisance of mosquitoes than with avoiding illness. This type of result has many implications for the promotional aspects of implementation. Problems with responses in health interviews are well recognized (Campbell et al. 1979; Kroeger 1985). Survey questions must be adapted and refined to ensure that they are appropriate for each application.

It will not be practical to do a baseline survey before every ITN project in every community, but the variables described below are important inputs for preparing the strategy. Key information can be collected using rapid-appraisal techniques.

What information is required from households?

Demographic profile

Listing members of each household generates the following variables, which should influence the choice of strategy and the details of implementation: household size and composition, the number of women and children in vulnerable age groups, the number of households headed by women, and the number of members who temporarily live elsewhere for work or school.

The concepts of "household" (husband and wife unit) and "homestead" (several households sharing a compound) are related but not identical. For example, average household size in West Kabar, Kenya, was 4.7 people (Hill 1990), whereas homesteads identified by the elders (*miji-kumi*) had 12.5 people on average (Feilden 1991). The Kilifi field trial uses the compound as the unit to which ITNs are issued; within each compound, one Bed Net Contact Person is identified (E.S. Some, personal communication). Using the larger group as the point of contact reduces contacts between clients and staff or community workers; this may save time but may also dilute the effectiveness of passing on essential messages.

Information about households headed by women can draw attention to potential constraints on traveling to services or on money for transport and services. These problems tend to be found where culture and male migration for work affect women's decision-making. These constraints must be assessed if equity is an objective of the intervention.

Mobile ITNs

Some ITN projects have found their calculations of supply requirements and monitoring of coverage complicated by migration of family members, who may take ITNs with them, and by visits from guests, who may occupy household ITNs. For example, about 5% of ITNs found during household surveys in Dar es Salaam bore indelible registration numbers from rural ITN projects (Evans 1994). In Papua New Guinea, the number of ITNs distributed did not reflect regular use by household members because new ITNs were kept for guests (Curtis et al. 1991). In Kenya, children take ITNs with them when they go away to school (Hill 1991).

The Bagamoyo project also found that mobile ITNs are needed. An ITN taken away by a migrant worker is not a lost investment, even if the intervention's primary target groups are pregnant women and small children. It could be argued that the mobile ITN increases the household's capacity to buy another ITN for dependents to use at home. The need for extra ITNs for family members who are temporarily resident elsewhere should be considered when planners are estimating quantities of supplies.

Buildings, beds, and bedding

It is important for planners to understand who sleeps where and what type of bedding is used when they are estimating the number and size of ITNs required or the number and type of nets to be treated. The importance of distinguishing between structures in the compound and structures used for sleeping was illustrated by a survey of Ovamboland, northwest Namibia (Meek and Kamwi 1991). The mean number of buildings per household was 12.1 (range 2–43), but the mean number of sleeping rooms was only 4.4 (range 1–13). Data from spraying projects, which are based on number of buildings, would give a serious overestimate of ITN requirements.

The first knowledge, attitudes, and practices survey for Kenya's Bamako Initiative projects indicated that each family-size net would be used by 2.5 people (husband, wife, and infant). This occupancy rate is still used (J. Hill, personal communication). A large project in Afghanistan and in refugee villages in Peshawar, Pakistan, also uses an occupancy rate of 2.5 people per net (S. Hewitt, personal communication). The baseline study for this project had found that people often moved beds outside and put two *charpoys* together, a sleeping arrangement also found in Bagamoyo, Tanzania.

The WHO/TDR Kilifi trial in Kenya counted structures in the compound and measured beds in detail. The average Kilifi bed is longer than a standard rectangular net, which is 180 cm long, and modern beds are larger overall (E.S. Some, personal communication). The dimension of interest is the perimeter (Table 7). The dimensions of two standard-size beds found in Dar es Salaam are also shown. What is needed for operational planning is a frequency distribution of the perimeters of

Table 7. Dimensions of beds in Kilifi, Kenya, and Dar es Salaam, Tanzania.

	Average width (cm)	Average length (cm)	Perimeter (cm)
Kilifi			
Traditional bed	96	183	670[a]
Modern bed	104	195	710[a]
Dar es Salaam			
Single bed	107	183	580
Double bed	152	183	670

Source: Kilifi — E.S. Some (personal communication); Dar es Salaam — Evans (1994).
[a] For Kilifi, this is average perimeter plus two standard deviations.

beds in use, including two single beds pushed together if this is the custom. Net size is discussed further in "Decisions About Bednets," pp. 77–86.

A small field trial in rural Cameroon found that 1 year after 400 ITNs were distributed, the mismatch between ITN size and bed size was so serious that 23 % of the nets were not installed and another 32 % were ripped. When asked about the inconvenient features of their nets, 41 % of respondents said they were too short or too small (Louis et al. 1992). Other studies found that bedding would tear a conventional net or would allow mosquitoes to enter from below (MacCormack et al. 1989).

Urban sleeping arrangements have been studied in planned and squatter settlements in Dar es Salaam. Men sleep outside from the age of 10. If someone is sleeping on a mat, the household puts a higher priority on buying a bed than on buying nets (Evans 1994).

The task of choosing the best fabric, design, and size for nets for an ITN project does not arise if people already use nets. Project workers would need to know what size nets are most common and, more important, what they are made of. The different absorbencies of cotton and synthetic fibres mean that if the net contains a mixture of fabrics, instructions for dipping must take this into account (see Chapter 2). Operational approaches for dealing with these complexities are discussed in a later section (see "Following a Recipe," pp. 101–102).

Preliminary investigation of sleeping spaces both inside and outside buildings should also establish whether it would be easier to hang a conical net (with one central hanging point) or a rectangular net. This information is also needed for promotional material that informs new users how to hang a bednet.

In some situations, bednets are not feasible. For example, a preliminary analysis of sleeping arrangements in rural Burkina Faso found that most women and children used huts that were too small for bednets. Instead, treated curtains were hung over doors, windows, and eaves (A. Habluetzel, personal communication).

Mosquito control

Many preliminary studies asked the householder about mosquito-control measures, and some tried to determine whether these measures were to reduce the nuisance of mosquitoes or to prevent malaria. Information about mosquito control is needed for directing promotional activities correctly (see Chapter 4) and for finding out whether current household expenditure could be diverted to ITNs (see "Spending Power," pp. 72–73).

Table 8. Multiple methods of mosquito control (% use) in Dar es Salaam, Tanzania.

	Households with nets (62% of sample)	Households without nets (38% of sample)
Net alone	38	0
Coils and sprays	13	10
Coils	34	64
Sprays	17	9
Nothing	0	16

Source: Evans (1994).

Data from Dar es Salaam (Table 8) showed that most urban households with untreated nets also used other methods of mosquito control (Evans 1994).

Where ITNs are used, they are not a complete substitute for other control methods, such as coils and aerosols, because people need protection during the evening before they get under the ITN. Also, households may not have enough ITNs to protect everyone (discussion in Mikocheni, Dar es Salaam, Evans 1994):

> Say you have three beds. You cover the smallest ones and yourself, but the rest go without and are the mosquitoes' food.

When a community-based health project in West Orcot, Kenya, first offered locally made nets for sale, teachers and health professionals — who might be considered social trendsetters — were the first to buy them (J. Miesen, personal communication). In households with a better physical infrastructure — sealable windows, ceiling boards, and electricity — electrically heated vaporizing mats, fans, screens, and air conditioning probably make an important contribution to mosquito control. The extent to which ITNs replace other forms of mosquito control, especially in poorer households, must be researched further.

What type of ITN is preferred?

Preliminary data collection can be used to assess preferences in size, style, and colour, which are discussed later in this chapter. Chapter 2 covers the technical details.

In the Bagamoyo intervention, rectangular nets in three different sizes were taken from house to house and shown to potential purchasers (Makemba et al. 1995). Kenya's malaria-control project dropped plans to offer two sizes of net, apparently to simplify procurement. In Afghanistan, one size of net was chosen that would cover two *charpoys* side by side; stocking a single size simplifies implementation and is cheaper per person covered (M. Rowland, personal communication). Experience from smaller projects in which net prices must cover costs shows that a variety of products will cater to different household budgets (C. Reed, personal communication). A larger profit margin on fancy styles can subsidize the basic model (J. Miesen, personal communication).

Washing ITNs

Where nets are already used, it is important to find out how often they are washed because laundering affects the residual insecticide severely. Surveys have found that some net owners prefer to wash them every 1 or 2 weeks as reported from Ecuador and Peru (Kroeger et al. 1995), Dar es Salaam (Evans 1994), and The Gambia (MacCormack and Snow 1986). However, householders' reports may exaggerate the frequency with which they wash their nets. This has been elegantly demonstrated from research in a Mandinka village in The Gambia, where 68% of people said they washed their nets once every 2 weeks. Using water-soluble ink as a marker, researchers monitored the villagers' nets, checking them once per week for 16 weeks. None of the 130 nets was washed as often as every 2 weeks: the mode (31%) was one wash in 16 weeks (Miller et al. 1995). The frequency distribution is shown in Figure 10.

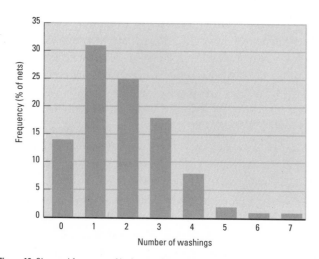

Figure 10. Observed frequency of bednet washing during a 16-week period in The Gambia (sample size = 130) (source: Miller et al. 1995).

In some field trials, nets have been distributed free of charge with instructions not to wash them for 6 months. These trials do not compare with programs where the users pay for their nets. Washing is sometimes necessary, for example, if a sick person has vomited on it. People who have bought their nets want them to be clean for various reasons: to avoid breathing the dust that collects on the net and to present a well-kept house. This "houseproud factor" has been eloquently described by focus groups in Dar es Salaam (Evans 1994):

> All nets are usually white, if you saw it dirty it doesn't look nice, and when you think that not only is this room a bedroom, it is also a sitting room when visitors come ...!
>
> When a visitor comes you'll be so ashamed if the net is hanging there filthy, all grey with dust and dirt from the children's fingers.
>
> ... so you'll have to wash it because visitors may come round and you don't want them to see the dirty net, do you?

The desire to keep nets looking pristine should not be underestimated when planners are choosing a strategy for treating them with insecticide. The association between washing frequency and net colour has not been studied among people who choose and purchase their own nets. The interaction between need to wash nets and choice of ITN strategy is discussed later in "Washing Bednets," (p. 105).

Uselife of nets

Where nets are already used, studies have tried to find out how long they last. For example, in 1985, in a Mandinka village where 154 people were interviewed, the uselife of locally made nets was estimated at 6 years; the fabric was not specified (MacCormack et al. 1989). On the coast of Ecuador, where 78% of nets were cotton mesh, uselife was 4.5 years, and in the Peruvian Amazon, where 93% of nets were cotton mesh, uselife was 3 years (Kroeger et al. 1995). Polyethylene nets were much more durable than polyester-fibre mesh in a field trial in rural Tanzania (C. Curtis, personal communication). In Dar es Salaam, surveys found that respondents' estimates of uselife (22–29 months) were affected by two factors: recall problems and the fact that some were using nets for the first time and had no experience of how long a net would last (Evans 1994).

In operational research, uselife is a variable needed for calculating the annual capital cost, which must be included in estimates of annual household expenditure on mosquito control (see also "Decisions About Bednets", pp. 77–86). The most reliable data are likely to come from long-term interventions, such as those in Afghanistan and Kenya, where net purchases are registered. The registers provide a database from which the uselife of nets with known characteristics (fabric, denier, and size) can be found. We assume that people want to know how long a net will last and how often it will need to be replaced. However, this aspect of decision-making has not been documented; for example, there might be a market for relatively inexpensive, flimsy, short-lived "guest nets."

Other information on knowledge, attitudes, and practices

The preliminary data collected from households can be used to assess knowledge of the malaria vector and attitudes toward preventing the disease. These findings should be used not only in designing health-education messages and materials but also in training health promoters, village-level workers, and health staff.

Study of knowledge, attitudes, and practices might help to identify in advance any barriers to using insecticide on nets. For example, Curtis (1992b) reported that in Sichuan Province, China, villagers who raise silkworms keep them in trays in their houses and were concerned that insecticide sprayed on bednets would harm the young silkworms. The recommendation was to avoid harm by removing the trays of young silkworms during spraying and to use a liquid formulation rather than a wettable powder (WP), presumably because WP tends to flake off and might fall into the silkworm trays after the treated net has dried.

Another example of a barrier to using ITNs has been encountered in Tanzania. Winch et al. (1993) described how whole families are occupied with a task that exposes them to mosquitoes during the local vector's feeding time:

> When the rice is maturing, people in Bagamoyo District migrate to their fields for several months, towards the end of the long rains, to guard the rice from birds, wild pigs, wart hogs and hippopotami. Birds are the major concern during the day, and frightening them off is often the responsibility of children. Pigs are the major concern at night, and they are guarded [against] either by adults alone, or by whole families .... Adults typically sleep on a bed or mat in the open on an elevated piece of ground.
> Using a net is inconvenient for [four] reasons:
> ❖ it is harder to see the pigs if one is inside a net;
> ❖ fire, especially torches, is used to drive off the animals. It is inconvenient and dangerous to have burning objects in the vicinity of a net;
> ❖ it is hard to suspend a net outside of a house; and
> ❖ sleeping under a net gives the pig a head start because it takes time to get out of the net.

Heat and stuffiness are sometimes given as reasons for not wanting to use an ITN. In rural Cameroon, 47 % of respondents mentioned heat as an inconvenient feature of nets after using them for 1 year (Louis et al. 1992). In Ghana, no one complained about heat after 3 months of use, but "they said they would erect poles on the roof to mount [the nets] during the hot season" (Gyapong et al. 1992).

Cost

Household expenditure on mosquito control has been assessed in several studies. Weekly and monthly expenditure on essentials and on luxuries (discretionary purchases) have also been assessed. If these data are to be used for policy decisions, such as how much people should be asked to pay for ITNs, nets, or insecticide treatment, three points must be considered.

First, the questions must be correctly formulated. In Yaoundé, Cameroon, two questionnaires designed to cover the same subject matter obtained vastly different information on whether anyone in the household had been ill on account of mosquitoes and on the amount spent on protection against mosquitos and treatment for mosquito-related illnesses. The first survey, in 1988, used suggestive wording and asked about expenditure without any details or consistency checks. By contrast, the 1990 questionnaire used a shorter recall period and removed the suggestion of malaria or mosquitoes from the wording of the question; only illness that incurred expenditure was counted. For the question about expenditure on protection and treatment, the 1990 survey built up the variables from many step-by-step questions that respondents could answer more accurately. Table 9 compares estimates of incidence for mosquito-related disease and expenditure on protection against mosquitoes and treatment for malaria from the two surveys (Louis et al. 1990). Expenditures on protection and treatment estimated from the 1988 survey were more than double those estimated from the 1990 survey.

Table 9. Two estimates of illness from mosquitoes and expenditure on protection and treatment, from Yaoundé, Cameroon.

| | | Annual expenditure ($) | | |
	Anyone ill on account of mosquitoes?	On protection	On treatment	Total
1988 (March)	40% in the last 15 days	105	233	338
1990 (February)	4.4% incurred expenditure in the last 7 days	65	93	158

Source: Louis et al. (1990).

The 1988 survey also seems to have overstated incidence of mosquito-related illness. The danger of unreliable estimates of household expenditure is that they may be used in developing strategies for promoting ITNs with unrealistic expectations of what people are able to pay.

Second, the distribution of expenditure (and disposable income) should be considered. Studies typically report average expenditure and average percentage of monthly income spent on protection from the nuisance of mosquitoes and on treatment costs. Occasionally, they also report the range and number of families not spending on particular types of mosquito control (for example, Guiguemde et al. 1994). From these statistics, it is clear that the distribution is skewed and that the mean is inflated by relatively few high-spending households. The average overstates current expenditure and ability to pay. Even where the highest income group spends more money on mosquito control than the lowest, this expenditure represents a smaller share of household income for the well-off group. In Dar es Salaam, high-income households spent 3.1% of declared income on all control methods; low-income households spent 7.4% (Evans 1994). In The Gambia, the average weekly household expenditure on discretionary items was $0.70, and ITN dipping would be considered a discretionary item; however, 25% of households reported no discretionary spending (S. Zimicki, personal communication). Equitable strategies cannot be developed without data on distribution of household expenditure; these data can be refined by identifying spending on staples, on luxuries, and on all items related to mosquitoes (control and treatment). This information would indicate how many people could afford to buy ITNs and how many would require subsidy or exemption.

Finally, ITNs are not a perfect substitute for all other forms of mosquito control (see also "Can Bednets Be Used?," p. 77, Chapter 4). Older children and adults are likely to be exposed to the vector for several hours during the evening, when they use coils or sprays. Household expenditure on mosquito control before bedtime must be considered when calculating the possibilities for diverting expenditure into ITNs.

Spending power

If users must pay part of the cost of ITNs, then spending patterns and decisions must be assessed to develop the structure of payments. Information about "willingness to pay" is unreliable because it is a response to a hypothetical question. Operational planning for a cost-covering or cost-recovery scheme needs information about two aspects of spending power: how much cash might be available for ITNs and at what seasons of the year, and who would make the decision to purchase a net or pay for an insecticide treatment. Knowing which member of the household decides whether to purchase an ITN or a dip helps to target health-education messages and promotional material. Knowing the seasonal pattern of cash flow would allow providers to make nets and dips available at those times of the year when cash is available, which may not coincide with the start of the malaria season. In Bagamoyo, payment for cash crops is received in January, whereas production of mosquito larvae peaks in May and childhood mortality peaks in July and August (Winch et al. 1994). The African Medical Research Foundation project in Tanzania has found that the months of the malaria season, April and May, are financially difficult; however, "it seems that the stimulus of serious malaria, related to the rains, is stronger than convenience" because net sales peaked during these months (C. Reed, personal communication).

Some aspects of spending power were discussed with respondents in Dar es Salaam (Evans 1994). Although 77% had never borrowed money, 76% said that they would borrow to buy a net. Respondents in squatter settlements, where the physical infrastructure is poor, were significantly more likely to say that they would borrow to buy a net than respondents in planned areas. Households that already owned a net were more likely to borrow so that they could buy another net than households without nets.

This study also described a form of traditional saving, known as *upatu*, that resembles a revolving credit scheme. Although some men regard *upatu* as a women's game for raising pocket money, key informants indicated that women use the scheme to save cash for family essentials that the male head of household will not pay for or for seed capital for small-business ventures. Sheik Hashim, quoted in Evans (1994), said

> From olden times women have had means of saving food or other resources for a rainy day. It is one way of existing in a world where nothing is certain. Women on the coast in big towns like Zanzibar, Pemba, Tanga, Mombasa, Malindi and Lamu had traditional ways of saving money that were called "Upatu." They have helped alot of women in times of trouble without them having to borrow money.

Upatu is specifically described as an urban phenomenon; in rural households, saving schemes are less likely to be cash based. The point to emphasize is that indigenous practices and current experience should be sought out before launching an ITN scheme that requires financial participation from the users.

What information can be gathered at the community level?

As with household surveys, experience of gaining insights from community leaders and key informants is well documented. This approach is probably easier in rural areas, where both the leaders and the boundaries of the community are usually well defined. Each country has its traditional and administrative structures, and the incumbents at community level should be included when developing strategies. In Bagamoyo, leaders of village governments were involved in selecting candidates for the village bednet committees, but this did not overcome indifference or animosity to the ITN intervention. The local leaders also complained that the village government's role in implementing ITN activities had not been specified. In the second phase of implementation, these local leaders were invited to the 1-day orientation seminar for members of the village bednet committee and were more actively involved in promoting net sales (Makemba et al. 1995).

Care should also be taken to include women, who have the main responsibility for looking after nets and getting them treated. Women's views about feasible strategies may differ from those put forward by men. Discussions should cover the following:

❖ Access by, for example, public transport;

❖ Seasonality, such as when roads are impassable, when people are totally occupied with their livelihood, and when cash is available;

❖ Commercial outlets and the products available;

❖ The range of socioeconomic conditions within the community;

❖ Village health workers and traditional birth attendants, who may be participating in the meeting, and local health services; and

❖ Ways of ensuring equity of access to ITNs.

Any aspect of involvement that may be required during implementation should be discussed with community representatives. For example, in Afghanistan, where access is constrained by severe winter weather, NGOs and mobile teams visit the village to notify the elders the day before nets and dipping are offered; the message is then broadcast from the mosques' loudspeakers.

Community views on "willingness to pay" and appropriate price structures must be handled with great care. Elders and official representatives are likely to be in a better financial position than some members of their community. Village health workers who periodically visit every household in their charge may have a better idea than local leaders of what families can afford. At a 2-week training workshop held for community health workers, traditional birth attendants, and village health committee members in Sigoti, Kisumu District in Kenya, participants were told that the community decides on the charges for nets and dipping and how to use the revenue — for example, on more permethrin, on making more local nets, or on any other project selected by the community. The next day, the following comment was recorded in the proceedings (GOK–UNICEF 1990):

> The net charge as designed by the VHC [Village Health Committee] is high, should be 50/- [Kenyan shillings] not 75/- .... Participants raised concern about the VHC verdict over the price of a net which was 75/- per net and redipping to be 7/50 per net per round. The participants said it's high and therefore called for more review.

As the members of the village health committee had set this price, it was presumably the community health workers and traditional birth attendants who thought the price was too high. They said that the coverage target might not be achieved because few people would buy at that price. Further on, the proceedings record that

> The Village Health Committee reviewed the charges and later came up with the table below:

Net	55/- [Kenyan shillings]
Redipping	10/-

In The Gambia, the system for collecting treatment fees (collection in advance in the village and a receipt for the number of nets to be treated) was set without being discussed with the potential customers. In 1993, in the areas where payment for treatment was introduced, 50% of households with nets paid for insecticide (S. Zimicki, personal communication), but in the eastern part of the country, coverage after the dipping fee was introduced was only 10% (Pickering 1993).

If a community financing scheme is to be used, careful preparations must be made for choosing people to handle money, keep records, and monitor bookkeeping and stock management. Anecdotal evidence from Papua New Guinea suggests that women are more reliable in local fund management than men. In Kenya, the Bamako Initiative projects suggest recruiting female treasurers to village health committees. This approach is not feasible in rural Afghanistan for cultural reasons, so the system is designed to monitor everything using written records of stock and transactions.

If nets and insecticide are to be supplied through the private sector, information about suitable outlets must be obtained at the community level. If nets are already available, the type, quality, and local market price should be ascertained.

What is needed from the health system?

According to Sexton (1993),

Where [primary health care] infrastructure exists, it should serve as the implementor of the net programme. Where it does not exist, PHC should be promoted, but other organisations should be sought to serve, until PHC becomes a reality .... The involvement of the PHC system especially at district and health centre level, is imperative for a sustainable programme.

The staff who will promote and provide ITN services in the government health system, NGOs, or employers' clinics will have to be trained. Preparation for training could include assessing their skills in explaining to clients how existing measures contribute to reducing transmission of malaria. If their role includes supporting and supervising community committees, they must be taught how to do these tasks, which may differ from their past activities.

If a government health service is to deliver the ITN program, its capacity to receive, store, and dispatch supplies and to transport them to the point of use must be assessed at both central and district levels. The assessment may show that major improvements in logistics and stock management are needed before valuable supplies can be consigned with confidence to the government's distribution system. Adding new items such as nets, insecticide, and mixing equipment to stock records is relatively straightforward; however, registering and reporting net sales or distribution and treatment of nets will require new formats, as will financial reporting.

Senior health managers should participate in developing an operational strategy so that it is not imposed from outside. In many hospitals, malaria is the most frequent diagnosis for both out-patients and in-patients and is a leading cause of death. In Kenya, some hospitals already sell ITNs (J.L. Hill, personal communication) and use nets that are specially designed for in-patients (C. Reed, personal communication). However, not all hospital managers are aware or convinced of the effectiveness of ITNs.

Decisions About Bednets

When the information described above has been obtained, it will be clear whether households are already using nets or can obtain them from local shops. If nets are not available at an affordable price, the intervenors face several decisions. This section concentrates on decisions that need to be made by those planning to procure or produce nets in bulk.

Can bednets be used?

The first question is whether local sleeping arrangements permit the use of bednets. Even if people sleep on the roof in hot weather, as they do in Ghana, or outside on beds or on the ground, as they do in Afghanistan, it is possible to arrange a net support. However, some houses are not suitable for bednets. This was the case in Burkina Faso, where the houses are very small and used for cooking, as well as for sleeping, and many things hang from the ceiling because there is nowhere else to store them. This prompted investigators in one large-scale trial to hang curtains over windows, doors, and eaves (A. Habluetzel, personal communication; Figure 11). Once it is established that bednets can be used, the choice has to be made from among a great variety of designs, fabrics, and sizes.

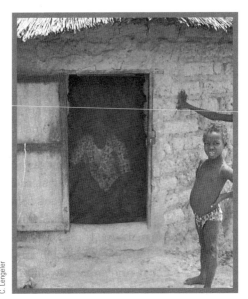

Figure 11. An insecticide-treated door curtain in Burkina Faso.

Sources of bednets

Where will nets be made or purchased?

❖ *homemade*: Some Ecuadorian households choose this option, which may work if the right material is available.

❖ *Tailored locally*: This work can be done by a professional tailor or by an existing group that also does other tasks. This option is especially attractive when the cost of netting is a barrier; recycled materials can also be used, as in Bénin (S.F. Rashed, personal communication).

❖ *Purchased ready made*: This option includes locally manufactured, imported, and second-hand nets.

❖ *Distributed through a project*: The project would decide whether to use a local manufacturer or commercial outlet or to procure from international sources.

Net design

The four basic net designs are rectangular, conical, A-frame, and triangular (Figure 12). To date, all donor-funded projects in Africa using imported nets have chosen rectangular ones (Figure 13). The surface area of a rectangular net is easy to measure for estimating the amount of insecticide required, and such a net will not sag across the edges of the bed. In Ecuador, most homemade nets are rectangular; they are easier to make and accommodate more people than conical nets because the four corners hold it off the occupants (Kroeger et al. 1991). However, the rectangular design is tailored to a specific bed size and will not stretch to fit a larger bed.

Conical nets hang from the centre and spread over a ring made of metal, wire, or cane or a frame of spokes (Figure 14). Some conical nets have a circular ceiling; others are gathered to the central hanging point. Some commercially manufactured conical nets, such as those made by Emnet in Zimbabwe, come in different sizes; others are advertised as one-size-fits-all. One-size nets are gathered at the top or from the ring to allow the spread of extra fabric required for fitting any bed. Gathering also adds to the elegant draped effect featured in some promotional material.

Users experienced with both rectangular and conical nets say that gathered nets sag, which is a problem if they are not treated because

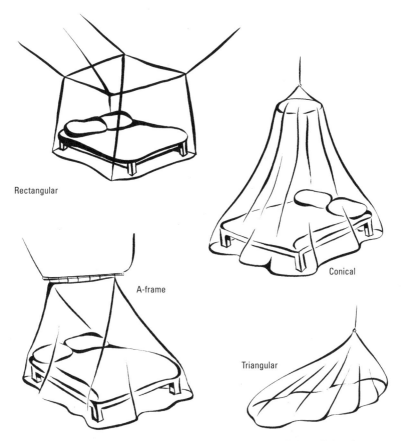

Figure 12. The four main types of net design: rectangular, conical, A-frame, and triangular.

mosquitoes bite through the net. Fitted conical nets sag much less. Clients of the community-based PHC scheme in West Pokot, Kenya, expressed a preference for round nets, so local tailors were taught how to make a conical net from rectangular pieces of material measuring 202 cm × 183 cm and a round piece for the ceiling (top of the net). The rectangles are cut and assembled as shown in Figure 15. The instructions indicate that all seams should be bound with pocketing material. Like a rectangular net, this conical model does not stretch and must be made in different sizes.

One manufacturer makes A-frame nets for travelers. They come with supports to suspend the net over any size of bed. This shape requires generous gathering along the single seam at the top. An ungathered

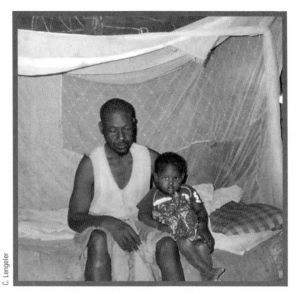

C. Lengeler

Figure 13. A rectangular net in The Gambia.

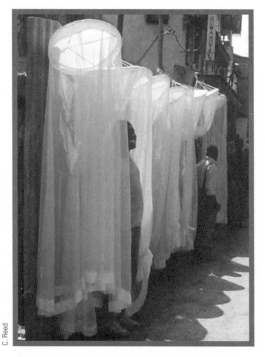

C. Reed

Figure 14. Conical nets for sale in Zanzibar market, Tanzania.

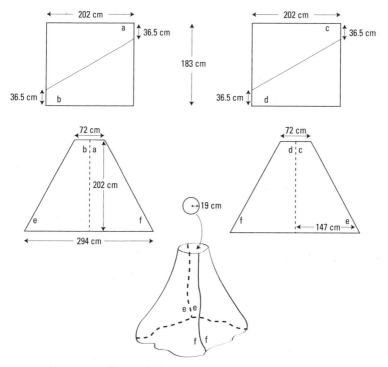

Figure 15. Sewing pattern for a fitted conical net.

A-frame net, called the "Turkana Tent," has been made for use in boarding schools (C. Reed, personal communication).

A triangular net is asymmetrical, with the apex of the net above the user's head. This type of net is used by some armed forces and has the advantages of small surface area, which makes it cheaper to make and to treat with insecticide, and low volume, which makes it more acceptable in small rooms (E.S. Some, personal communication). The Kilifi trial found that people do not like using a net if it takes up more than 40% of the room's volume (E.S. Some, personal communication).

Special features can be added to the basic model. The ceiling of a rectangular or conical net can be made of heavier material. A border can be added around the bottom of the net for tucking under rough bedding or weighting the net so that it touches the ground. Nets can also be weighted with a casing filled with pebbles (Emnet Rukukwe™). A net can also have an elasticized bottom edge so that it pulls close under the mattress (Emnet Paradise™). "Doors" can be let into a net with overlaps at least 60 cm wide.

Size and surface area

Net specifications are based on the bed size or sleeping space to be covered. Table 10 gives the dimensions of rectangular nets with two standard bed sizes found in Dar es Salaam (Evans 1994) for comparison. The nets are arranged according to the length of the lower perimeter, in ascending order. This dimension indicates whether the net would be able to cover a particular bed.

The largest custom-made rectangular net, a special order for the project in Afghanistan, was designed to cover two traditional single beds pushed together. The lower perimeters of the double conical nets (fitted and gathered) are longer than that of the largest rectangular net.

The largest ready-made rectangular net (X-family) is not too large when compared with data on the average bed on the Kenyan coast. The preliminary fieldwork in Kilifi found that bednets measuring 200 × 150 × 170 cm would fit most beds (Snow et al. 1993), but the nets ordered were 190 × 180 × 150 cm (the standard X-family size) (E.S. Some, personal communication). The lower perimeter of the net could fit around the average bed, but 5% of the nets were too small.

The width in which netting is manufactured must be considered when choosing design and size. The knitting machines at SiamDutch, for example, make fabric 300 cm wide (M. Dubbelman, personal communication).

Table 10. Dimensions, surface area, and lower perimeter of some nets, with dimensions of two beds for comparison.

Size	Width (cm)	Length (cm)	Height (cm)	Area (m²)	Perimeter[a] (cm)
Nets					
Single	70	180	150	8.8	500
Double	100	180	150	10.2	560
Single fitted conical	123	183	—	8.6	612
Family	130	180	150	11.6	620
A-frame, gathered top	184	184	198	14.6	736
X-family	190	180	150	14.5	740
Widest family	220	180	150	16	800
Double fitted conical	274	183	—	12.5	914
Double gathered conical (with door)	—	—	250	23	1 250
Beds					
Small	107	183	—	—	580
Large	152	183	—	—	670

[a] Perimeter = 2 × (width + length).

Choosing a net height of 150 cm — half the fabric width — means that no material is wasted, keeping costs to a minimum.

In the Bagamoyo project, nets were available in three sizes, but in the first distribution, people complained that they did not get the right size. Village bednet committee members did not carry all three sizes when they went from house to house evaluating requirements. If they saw single beds, they recommended single nets, not realizing that the householder needed a larger net to cover two single beds pushed together (Makemba et al. 1995).

Gathered conical nets are far more difficult to size and are generally sold by bed size (cot, bunk, single, three-quarter, double, queen, or king) or by width.

Surface area is important because of its cost implications for insecticide treatment. Table 10 shows that for a given type of fabric, the largest net has three times the surface area of the smallest net and, therefore, will take three times more insecticide. A rectangular net with a 60-cm door has an extra 0.9 m² of surface area. Fitted conical nets cover the greatest area of bed with the smallest surface area of net.

Netting

When specifying mesh material or buying mesh to make nets, three choices must be made (see Chapter 2):

- ❖ *Fibre*: May be natural (cotton) or synthetic (polyester, nylon, or polyethylene). It is usually difficult to find out what fibres a non-project net contains.

- ❖ *Denier*: Indicates the strength of the thread and is defined by the weight in grams of 9 000 m of thread. Nets are typically made of 40-, 75-, or 100-denier threads. The strongest thread is 100 denier, and this is recommended because it survives the inevitable wear and tear longest and is only a little more expensive. Polyethylene is more durable than mesh made from synthetic fibre, but consumer preferences for synthetics or polyethylene have not been tested in interventions in Africa.

- ❖ *Mesh*: Is defined by the number of holes per square inch; thus, 156 mesh has 156 holes (12 × 13), and 196 mesh has 196 holes (14 × 14). The wider mesh, 156, is effective for bednets and allows more ventilation.

If nets are made of other fabrics, the choice is limited only by the market and personal preference. For example, the opaque draperies used around beds in many parts of The Gambia not only prevent mosquito bites but also provide privacy, warmth, and protection from dust (and from unwelcome wildlife, such as snakes) (MacCormack et al. 1989).

Colour

There seem to be two conflicting preferences: in some places, white nets are preferred because they look fresh and clean (see "Washing Bednets," p. 105) (J. Hill, personal communication); in others, ITNs cannot be kept clean if they must not be washed for 6 months. The TDR trial in Ghana found that white nets get dirty very quickly because nets are tucked under mats on the floor, children urinate on them, and the harmattan winds are strong (Gyapong et al. 1992). This important point was elicited during focus group discussions:

> These findings were elicited by the indirect way people spoke. For example, someone said, "It is just because it has been given to us white we cannot say anything bad, but if it were black it would have been better because with the winds the white gets dirty ...."

In response, the project distributed rust-coloured nets (F.N. Binka, personal communication), which were popular. Mesh colour affects operational planning because some manufacturers charge more for coloured nets (for example, 10% more for pastels and 20% more for dark colours, Table 11).

Table 11. Cost of project bednets in 1993/94, showing sources of variation in prices.

	X-family net	Sources of variation
Basic price from manufacturer	$4.06–4.50	+ 10% for pastels + 20% for dark colour + $0.40 for special size
International transport	5–30%	Distance to destination Sea freight cheaper than air freight
Tax	0–20%	Local policies
Clearance, demurrage, storage	Variable	Local administrative practices
Local transport	<1–2%	Distance to destination
Total cost, DDP	$4.54–5.65	Based on actual DDP prices

Note: DDP, delivered, duty paid.

Insecticide requirements

Generally, the amount of insecticide required to treat a net depends on

❖ Its surface area;

❖ The thickness of its fibre; and

❖ The type of fibre (cotton needs more insecticide than synthetics).

Once the amount of pure insecticide has been determined, the dipping solution must be prepared. Preparing the insecticide solution is the most difficult operational issue and a constant source of errors. Chapter 2 describes how to measure the absorptive capacity of a net before treating it so that insecticide and water can be mixed in the correct proportions.

The problems of treating nets of differing absorptive capacities in mixed batches have arisen only in interventions where people were already using a variety of nets. These problems have been addressed in Ecuador and the Solomon Islands by preparing dipping recipes for each type of net according to fabric and size.

Cost

Intervenors planning to provide nets must compare the full cost of obtaining them with the price of comparable nets in local commercial outlets. The full cost, known as DDP (delivered, duty paid), may include the following four components:

❖ *Basic price*: The cost from the manufacturer. Nets are usually cheaper in bulk than in small quantities; for example, SiamDutch quotes a price for a 20-foot (6-m) container of 25 000–30 000 pieces. Bulk procurement can save money.

❖ *Transport*: Charges for carriage, insurance, and freight (CIF) for nets imported by sea or air. Prices quoted as CIF cover the basic price plus transport and insurance to the port of destination. Prices quoted as free on board (FOB) only cover transport from the manufacturer to the port of shipment. Additional transport, incurring further charges, will be involved from that port to the final destination

❖ *Taxes*: Duty may be levied on imported nets, and value-added tax and sales tax may apply to commercial sales.

❖ *Clearance, demurrage, and storage*: Fees for customs clearance of imported nets. If unloading is delayed, the buyer may be charged demurrage, and if the goods are delayed in customs, the buyer may be charged for storage.

Several programs have provided basic prices and additional costs. Table 11 summarizes these data to indicate the basic costs and sources of variation, assuming that an ITN project is buying X-family rectangular 156-mesh nets in white 100-denier polyester. Projects reported DDP prices ranging from $4.54 to $5.65.

Although it is simple to obtain a CIF price quotation from a manufacturer, the costs of clearing goods through customs can be unpredictable. This uncertainty may affect small projects more seriously than large international donors. Data from Kenya and Tanzania indicate DDP costs are 25–33% of the price of nets in commercial outlets. (This calculation excludes administrative costs to the ITN project.)

Projects that make their own nets locally from imported mesh have found that fabric costs account for up to 70% of production costs, depending on net size. A design that minimizes surface area reduces costs (S.F. Rashed, personal communication). In cash-poor rural communities, locally tailored nets can be bartered for other assets, such as livestock (C. Reed, personal communication).

A more relevant indicator than the cost of the net may be the cost per person covered. With reliable data on how many people actually use nets and how long they last, the cost of net protection per person per year could be calculated and amortized at a positive discount rate. This calculation was done for the Government of Kenja (Ministry of Health)–UNICEF program in Kenya (Feilden 1991). The concept of amortization could be useful in developing price structures (see "Decisions About Financing," pp. 90–97).

Conclusion

The main equipment for this intervention — a mosquito net — comes in an enormous variety of forms. It is the major investment in ITN programs, so operational research to identify the important aspects of design, quality, and durability seems essential. For example, analysis of rips and tears should indicate whether different sizes and shapes would make the net last longer. No large intervention that supplies subsidized ITNs has been running for more than 5 years — frequently assumed to be the uselife of a net. Firm information on this variable is needed so that ITNs can be replaced in an orderly way.

Decisions About Insecticide

Synthetic pyrethroids

Synthetic pyrethroids (SPs) are the only insecticides currently used for treated nets. The three commonly used SPs are permethrin, deltamethrin, and lambdacyhalothrin. Chapter 2 covers the technical details of these insecticides and their safety.

No clear technical guidelines on SPs currently exist. As a result, a manufacturer was able to describe permethrin wettable powder as suitable for net treatment without demonstrating that it would stay on the net. A donor-funded intervention covering several districts bought this product, which is still in use, although the donor was informed that wettable powder is not suitable for ITNs because it falls off the fibres. This example suggests that a clearing centre for information on insecticides for ITNs is needed.

Public-health clearance

From an operational perspective, the first question is whether a pyrethroid is registered in the country for treating mosquito nets. Lack of this legal requirement has held back ITN schemes in Zimbabwe (T. Freeman, personal communication). Clear technical information prepared for non-specialist decision-makers would facilitate discussion with bureaucrats and politicians about the benefits of ITNs and the safety of the recommended insecticides.

Emphasizing the merits of ITNs should be part of any strategy to reduce financial barriers imposed by import duties and delays in customs clearance. ITN experience to date indicates that the effect of these barriers is probably underestimated because the largest interventions have been funded by international agencies that have privileged tax status, which permits them to expedite goods through customs. Small projects are less likely to have such privileges. Strategies are needed to improve local procedures for clearing valuable products that offer both commercial opportunities and public-health improvements. Essential drug programs offer some useful experience.

Sources

The three major insecticide producers (Zeneca, AgrEvo, and Sumitomo) all offer public-health-grade SPs formulated as emulsifiable concentrates

(ECs). All the brands seem equally effective for treating nets (see Chapter 2). The criteria for product selection, therefore, are availability (local or international), response time in providing a price quotation, reliability of supply, and technical support in answering queries.

Commercial availability varies from country to country, and a chosen pyrethroid may not be locally available (M. Rowland, personal communication). Local suppliers have been known to deliver agricultural pyrethroids for ITN use; such a delivery also occurred with one international procurement for an ITN trial. The procurement service of UNICEF Copenhagen does not list public-health pyrethroids in its catalogue. Most buyers for public-health programs do not know as much about pyrethroids as researchers running field trials, and inappropriate products are sometimes chosen. An information clearing house would help nonspecialist buyers choose suitable products and avoid wasting money on the wrong formulation.

Presentation

Chapter 2 covers effective ingredients, concentration, formulation, and packaging. Choices should be informed by both operational requirements and cost considerations. The total volume of a shipment is likely to be lower in 20-L drums than in 1-L bottles, implying lower costs of transport, storage, and handling. At point of use, however, a 20-L drum would be practical only if very large numbers of nets could be assembled and dipped at one site, for example, an urban dipping service. In most settings, 1-L bottles are more convenient because they obviate the need to pour insecticide from drums into smaller containers, which would also have to be supplied, incurring extra costs.

The weakest permethrin concentrate (10% EC) is more than five times bulkier per dose of insecticide than the 55% EC presentation. The most concentrated insecticide (lambdacyhalothrin) might be the least expensive to transport and store, but the costs associated with wastage from dilution errors are potentially greater.

Some programs have changed the insecticide concentration they use (for example, from 20% EC to 25% EC). The Afghanistan project has changed the insecticide itself from permethrin to lambdacyhalothrin for reasons of cost. The operational implication of changing either the concentration or the type of insecticide is that field staff must be thoroughly briefed, supervised, and monitored to ensure that the correct dosage is used.

Cost of insecticide

Transport costs are so variable that a factory-gate or FOB price is a poor indicator of the CIF price; therefore, manufacturers want to know the destination of the goods before quoting a price. When the price is quoted as supply call forward, shipping costs are estimates. Importation means further charges at customs. Table 12 summarizes some recent data from projects and programs that import permethrin, deltamethrin, and lambdacyhalothrin. The variable of interest is the annual cost of insecticide for treating one net; this variable appears in the last column of Table 12 for a double net (15 m^2), assuming that the desired dose of permethrin is 500 mg/m^2, of deltamethrin is 25 mg/m^2, and of lambdacyhalothrin is 20 mg/m^2. Only one dip of lambdacyhalothrin is needed per year (Curtis et al. 1994).

If destination is held constant, these data show that

❖ Airfreight costs 14–48% more than seafreight; and

Table 12. Cost of insecticide in 1993/94 in different presentations and cost per treated net.

	% EC	Size	Terms	Per litre	Per ITN of 15 m^2	Per year (required dips)
Dar es Salaam, Tanzania						
Permethrin	55	20 L	CIF	31.70	0.43	0.86 (2)
Kilifi, Kenya						
Permethrin by sea	25	25 L	DDP	11.00	0.33	0.66 (2)
Permethrin by air	55	20 L	DDP	35.88	0.49	0.98 (2)
Nairobi, Kenya						
Permethrin by sea	25	25 L	SCF	12.42	0.37	0.74 (2)
Permethrin by air	25	25 L	SCF	14.04	0.42	0.84 (2)
Accra, Ghana						
Permethrin	55	20 L	CIF	32.80	0.45	0.90 (2)
	50	1 L	CIF	27.00	0.41	0.82 (2)
	55	15 mL	CIF	106.67	1.60	3.20 (2)
Deltamethrin	2.5	20 L	CIF	36.01	0.54	1.08 (2)
	2.5	15 mL	CIF	117.33	1.76	3.52 (2)
Afghanistan						
Permethrin by air	25	1 L	DDP	16.84	0.51	1.02 (2)
West Africa						
Lambdacyhalothrin	2	1 L	FOB	154.50	0.46	0.46 (1)

Note: See text for details of treatment doses. CIF, carriage, insurance, and freight; DDP, delivered, duty paid; EC, emulsifiable concentrate; FOB, free on board; ITN, insecticide-treated net; SCF, supply call forward.

❖ Insecticide packed in 15-mL sachets is three to four times more expensive per ITN than the same insecticide in bulk (this cost difference is expected to diminish as sales volume of sachets rises).

These variations indicate that buyers should obtain several price quotes before ordering insecticide.

The easiest way to compare insecticide costs is a spreadsheet using

❖ Cost per volume for a standard EC formulation of the chosen insecticide;

❖ Target dose;

❖ Surface area of an individual net; and

❖ Number of treatments per year.

Chapter 2 covers variations in target doses for different fabrics. In Table 12, we used 500 mg/m² for permethrin, 25 mg/m² for deltamethrin, and 20 mg/m² for lambdacyhalothrin. Using permethrin at 200 mg/m² would cut the cost of a permethrin dip by 60%; similarly, using deltamethrin at 15 mg/m² would cut the cost by 40%. It should be noted that it is not always necessary to dip nets twice per year in areas where malaria is seasonal, as in The Gambia. Lambdacyhalothrin is the most persistent pyrethroid, and nets treated with it need dipping only once per year unless they are frequently washed. At a dose of 10 mg/m², an annual dip with lambdacyhalothrin costs $0.23 and is cheaper than two dips per year with permethrin at 200 mg/m².

Decisions About Financing

Financing policies

Once nets and insecticide are selected, who will pay for the ITNs? Financing policies can be any combination of market price, cost price, or subsidy for nets or insecticide, or both. Table 13 shows financing policies used by current ITN schemes.

ITN interventions offer two valuable products, one of which is not widely available through the private sector: so far, insecticide is not sold through commercial outlets, even in large towns. Projects and programs that provide ITNs do not want these investments to be recycled through private traders for profit; so, for the foreseeable future, financing and

Table 13. Examples of ITN programs and their financing.

Nets	Insecticide	Location and strategy
Household pays full cost; nets made locally	Provided by ITN program at subsidized prices	The Gambia — three methods of insecticide distribution (VHWs, MCH clinics, shops) in two presentations (bulk, sachet)
Household pays full cost; nets made at home or by local tailors	Provided by government free of charge	Sichuan, China — 2.34 million treated nets (3.85 million people)
		In some countries in South America — resources may be transferred from house spraying to net impregnation
Price paid by household covers production cost; profit margin controlled; local design in two sizes	Project sells at cost	Benin and other community-based projects — nets made locally; costs are kept low through bulk purchase of materials
Household pays subsidized price for nets, which are imported or manufactured locally; bought from the CHW through community pharmacy; one style, colour, and size	Provided through health service at subsidized price	Kenya's Bamako Initiative projects — aimed at communities meeting criteria including high mortality and morbidity and weak infrastructure; donor support includes funding, procurement, and developing management, including community pharmacies
Household pays subsidized price for nets, which are imported or manufactured locally; sales are through fixed clinics run by NGOs; mobile teams cover areas with no clinics	Provided free by project; net owner dips net under supervision; fee is being pilot tested	Afghanistan — nets are a novelty; project must inform and motivate sales; access is difficult, and services must be well advertised in advance; teams visit elders, who arrange announcements
Household buys from commercial outlet	Bought at commercial outlet	None at present — intervention arranges for supplies to reach the market; profit margins are left to the discretion of traders
Free (or heavily subsidized) distribution at health facilities for high-risk groups (newborns and pregnant women)	Free treatment for high-risk groups	Not yet tried — external (donor) support necessary

Note: CHW, community health worker; ITN, insecticide-treated net; MCH, mother and child health; NGO, nongovernmental organization; VHW, village health worker.

treatment fees will probably remain under the control of those implementing the programs.

Most of the ITN schemes listed in Table 13 are less than 5 years old. For the model involving seed capital and revolving funds, the long-term transition to financial sustainability must be evaluated.

One strategic choice to be made is whether ITN interventions will be integrated with other activities or kept separate. Where ITN accounts are consolidated with other transactions, as at the community pharmacy in Kenya's Bamako Initiative projects, the financial status of ITNs alone is difficult to assess, and failure to generate revenue from other items may jeopardize the whole scheme. This happened in the community-based project in West Pokot, where bakery losses concealed the financial feasibility of ITNs (J. Miesen, personal communication).

The need for a detailed review of financing strategies is discussed at the end of this section. The following points are highlighted from material on the operational aspects of implementation.

Price structures

Deciding on the price

Most ITN interventions that require users to pay at least something for the net or the treatment are prepared to make a large investment in subsidizing those supplies to promote the technology. The level of initial subsidy must be appropriate to the disposable income of the target market, and data on household expenditure, spending decisions, and their seasonality are crucial in making sound decisions. In noncash economies, sustainability requires complementary interventions, such as developing a barter market for ITNs or generating cash income. If nets are available in local shops, it is also important to set the subsidized price at a level compatible with market prices.

For Afghanistan, the following advice was given by M. Rowland (personal communication):

> When pitching the promotional price be careful: too low and the nets will be resold in the market place the next day, too high and you and your donors may be misled into thinking the project has failed (due to low uptake). Restrict the number of nets each household can buy to avoid reselling.

Reselling has occurred in Burundi and the Central African Republic, where a high subsidy resulted in the rapid disappearance of many nets from the distribution area (Van Bortel et al. 1996; A. Boner, personal communication). In The Gambia, all insecticide was provided free of charge until 1992; the next year, 221 PHC villages began charging $0.50 for treatment. In 53 villages, the *Alkalo* (headman) and *Imam* (religious leader) were asked to advise on the minimum and maximum amount that compounds might be willing to pay for insecticide. The cost of insecticide needed to treat the average number of nets in a compound exceeded the respondents' estimates of the maximum amount that compounds would be willing to pay by between 1.2 and 9 times, depending on the area (Mills et al. 1994). This study raised several issues regarding payment options.

❖ Should the villages decide how to raise funds or should fund-raising mechanisms be decided for them? The survey identified great variety in villages' experience of collective fund-raising and noted that some villages would find it difficult to agree on a mechanism.

❖ Should households with nets pay for the insecticide or should it be paid for by other means (such as a collective activity) that might involve contributions from people without nets, who would not benefit from the insecticide?

❖ When should the payment be made?

Managers of the National Impregnated Bednet Programme (NIBP) did not think that it would be feasible for its staff to collect payments from individual households. It was decided to send NIBP staff to collect funds for insecticide from villages at the end of harvest. Villagers would decide how to collect the money and would receive vouchers indicating the number of treatments paid for. There would be further opportunity to pay just before dipping. This advance payment scheme was tried, but at most, only half the net owners paid for treatment. Lack of money was given as a reason for not treating nets by 50% of surveyed households that had not treated their nets (S. Zimicki, personal communication). In the eastern part of the country, only about 10% of net owners paid for insecticide in advance (Pickering 1993). Some women hoped that if they refused to pay they would be given free insecticide; this emphasizes the difficulty of altering the terms under which insecticide is provided. Others wanted to get what they were paying for at the time of payment but were prevented from doing so because

❖ Insecticide was available in the villages for only a short time;

❖ Some village health workers would allow dipping on only 1 day; and

❖ Village politics prevented some families from participating in the dipping.

Net owners — the potential customers — do not seem to have been involved in the decision about how payment should be made.

In Kenya, the Bamako Initiative project did not start as a research project. From the beginning, it has taken the view that in the interests of sustainability, neither nets nor insecticide would be distributed free of charge. This pricing strategy has the advantage of sending a clear message that the ITN intervention involves two products, each of which has a price. The policy is that communities set prices with guidance from divisional health staff under supervision from PHC staff at district level. This guidance ensures that the price structure covers the costs of replacement stock for the community pharmacy.

When the pilot phase started in 1990, participants at the second workshop for training community health workers asked village health committee members to reduce the price of nets and to increase the price of dipping. The new pricing strategy of subsidizing the nets with higher insecticide prices takes account of the fact that people find it easier to pay relatively small amounts twice a year than to come up with one large sum. The extent of this cross-subsidy must be evaluated to assess the long-term sustainability of the pricing structure. Cross-subsidization between nets and dips can work as long as cheaper insecticide does not appear on the market. If it does, the ITN project will not be able to ensure that people who purchased project nets are also buying project insecticide.

Currently, nets bought from the Bamako Initiative projects cost $3.30–4.20, and a dip costs $0.50 (J. Hill, personal communication). Nets bought through the project cost one-fifth of the price in commercial outlets ($18) when the intervention began. The donors pay very low prices because they purchase in bulk and import under preferential conditions, which reduces all costs incurred between arrival of the shipment in port and delivery to the warehouse.

Evidence already cited shows that the price of insecticide is a barrier to ITN use (for example, Pickering 1993; S. Zimicki, personal communication). Therefore, the cheapest effective dose must be chosen (see Chapter 2 and "Cost of Insecticide," pp. 89–90).

Micro-credit and loans

When a lump-sum payment for a net is still too much for some households to afford, loans seem attractive. Experience of ITN loan schemes is limited. The community-based scheme in West Pokot had to stop allowing loans because of difficulty collecting the money once people had the net (J. Miesen, personal communication). However, people already buying mosquito-control products such as coils and sprays, who start paying for an ITN by instalments and are not allowed to take possession until the whole amount is paid, will still be buying coils and sprays to protect themselves from mosquitoes and will not get the benefit of their partially paid-for ITN (Evans 1994).

Promoting the benefits of ITNs and savings schemes, such as *upatu* in Dar es Salaam, seems to be a more promising approach. Savings groups are highly specific to particular communities or work groups (Mills et al. 1994). If an ITN project wanted to introduce a rotating savings and credit association, the salient features, such as amount and frequency of contributions and management of accounts, would have to be adapted to the individual community. For further information, see Geertz (1962), Ardener (1978), Bouman (1978), Miracle et al. (1980), and Ardener and Burman (1995).

Equity and exemptions

Can a pricing structure be designed to meet the objective of equity? How should exemptions be dealt with? One function of community-based schemes is to decide locally how to use resources to help households that are so poor that they can never participate in an ITN scheme unless they are exempt from paying. Exemptions must be funded from surplus revenue, which means setting fees high enough to cover all costs including exempt households and low enough to stimulate sufficient sales to generate the revenue. The ways that individual communities have addressed equity must be evaluated by talking to community ITN decision-makers, nonusers, and any users for whom the community has provided a free or subsidized net.

An alternative is to rely on subsidy from an external source (government or donor), and the implications of this must be clearly defined before the start of the program.

Financial management and monitoring

Having chosen a pricing structure, the details of organizing and managing finances must be developed. If the ITN project will manage the finances, a great deal of community-level work will be involved: this should be allowed for in project planning.

Time of payment

Will clients pay in advance or at the time of service? Who will collect the cash? Will receipts and countersignatures be used? The advance-payment strategy in The Gambia was intended to be more convenient both for the program (so that workers are not responsible for money and insecticide at the same time) and for the community (with payment made when cash is available). However, advance payment was not popular with the clients and discouraged participation. Similar reluctance to pay for ITNs in advance has been noted among Bagamoyo farmers, whose reservations were based on experience with the cashew marketing board, which issued receipts instead of cash for their crop and then paid late and sometimes not in full (Makemba et al. 1995). Some projects that tried to coordinate payment with periods when cash is available have found that sales rise when households perceive the need for nets, even though cash is short at that time of year (C. Reed, personal communication).

Who holds the money?

It would seem obvious that only reliable people should be entrusted with collecting fees and managing funds. Projects and programs tend not to publicize the embarrassments they have suffered through mishandling of this aspect of operations. Anecdotal evidence indicates that the national program in Papua New Guinea found women to be far more dependable in handling ITN receipts than men. The Bamako Initiative projects' planning and implementation guidelines state that it is preferable to choose a woman as village health committee treasurer and repeat this statement when discussing management at community level (Liambila et al. 1994). In the Bagamoyo field trial of seven villages, each village bednet committee holds its funds in a separate bank account. In Kenya's Bamako Initiative projects, all payment vouchers must be signed by the treasurer or secretary of the village health committee and the chair, as well as the recipient.

At village level, "community monitoring," through which social pressure exerts a restraining and directive influence, can be invoked. The trap to avoid is entrusting funds to the most powerful local person, whom the rest of the community would find it difficult if not impossible to monitor and challenge.

Paperwork

The project in Afghanistan provides ITNs through a variety of staff from mobile teams and different NGOs' static clinics, where they sell nets far from the gaze of headquarters. M. Rowland (personal communication) suggests the following:

> When valuable commodities like bednets are involved, monitor everything: implementors, buyers, your store, clinics, even the monitors themselves. Have as many checks in the system as possible: i.e., sales registers for implementors, corresponding revenue registers for the accountant, registers for the NGOs, for re-impregnations, receipt books showing individual purchasers and signatures, quality control of stocks and revenue.

Formats must be designed for easy use by both the primary user and supervisors, who must cross-check documentation. The training manual on financial management for district and divisional health-management teams in Kenya (GOK–UNICEF 1992) illustrates the paperwork developed for the Bamako Initiative projects. Guidelines for running the financial aspects of ITN programs take time to develop and must be revised on the basis of field experience over several years. Research trials are a useful source for such material only if financial sustainability is a specific objective tested over time, especially with respect to sustainable levels of supervision (that is, what would happen without the research team backstopping this process). Guidelines, working documents, and formats used by field staff in ITN projects should be assembled and reviewed.

Conclusion

Good decisions about financing are crucial to the health of an ITN project. Experience with this vast problem is expanding rapidly as more interventions incorporate some form of payment by clients (for example, Bennett and Ngalande-Banda 1994). Financial aspects of ITN projects, including price sensitivity among nonusers and users, need to be evaluated systematically and in detail.

Management Systems for Supply of Goods and Services

The systems required for operating a program or providing a service are referred to as logistics. Here, the specific aspects of management are distinguished.

Procurement

Large orders can usually be obtained at lower unit cost. Estimating the quantities needed in the long term is a skilled task; useful guidance is available in *Managing Drug Supply* (Management Sciences for Health 1981). Substantial savings may be achieved by procuring through agents who negotiate bulk contracts with manufacturers or suppliers.

In Africa, nets can be purchased from two manufacturers: Sunflag Ltd in Arusha, Tanzania, and Emnet Corp. in Zimbabwe. To date, however, most projects in Africa have used nets imported from Thailand.

Pipelines

A review of experience with ordering supplies shows that the pipelines (time elapsed between placing an order and receiving the goods) for nets and insecticide can be very long. Orders must be placed in good time to avoid stock-outs that would hold up the intervention.

In The Gambia in 1992, three separate orders of permethrin took 2–3 months to arrive (NIBP 1993b). In Kilifi, Kenya, permethrin took 8 weeks to come by airfreight — 6 weeks to Nairobi and 2 weeks for clearance and delivery to the project (E.S. Some, personal communication). Nets took nearly 4 months — 2 weeks from the manufacturers to the docks in Bangkok, 10 weeks at sea, and 4 weeks for clearance through Mombasa and delivery to Kilifi (Snow et al. 1993). In Afghanistan, permethrin airfreighted to Peshawar took 5 months to reach the project, even with the United Nations High Commission for Refugees as the intermediary. The previous consignment was held at customs for 4 months (M. Rowland, personal communication).

Seafreight takes longer but costs less than airfreight. Transport costs are based on a complex combination of volume (bulk), weight, and status — special handling for rush orders costs more. Therefore, programs can cut costs by planning ahead. They may also be able to negotiate better rates after monitoring freight charges; some immunization programs have discovered that substantial cost savings can be achieved by choosing the shippers, rather than allowing the supplier to do so. In Kilifi, transport by sea added 5.6% to the cost of the nets and 2.5% to the cost of the insecticide.

Shelf life

Insecticide should remain potent for at least 2 years if stored in a cool, dark place. Given the length of the pipeline, it may be important to specify a maximum age of insecticide at the time of dispatch. This stipulation will minimize the risk that it might lose potency while in storage. In one program, stock stored in hot conditions for 1 year was visibly different from a newly arrived batch of the same product (F. Pagnoni, personal communication). Loss of potency in storage can be minimized by refining methods for estimating the required quantities.

Stock management, supply, and distribution

The manual *Managing Drug Supply* (Management Sciences for Health 1981) addresses stock management, supply, and distribution issues. Some additional points should be raised, however, for ITN programs.

Where will stocks be stored? If they are in central medical stores, will they be distributed with other supplies? Is there storage space? Is the transport system from centre to periphery reliable and frequent enough for supplies to be distributed on time? Can the seasonality of use be managed within a regular quarterly or monthly distribution of supplies? Does the drug storage and supply system work well enough to be entrusted with nets and insecticide?

If a separate storage and distribution system is chosen, how will its staff salaries and running costs be funded? Does the workload justify a parallel storage and distribution system? How will transport costs — vehicles, as well as fuel and drivers — be funded?

Choice of presentation should take into account the practicalities of distributing insecticide to progressively smaller units. For example, the 1992 treatment coordinators in The Gambia noted that distribution bottlenecks were caused by mistakes in the quantities of containers and markers packed at the central store and by a shortage of 5-L containers, which were unavailable in the markets. This program procures insecticide in 20-L drums that must be split into smaller quantities; 5 L is considered the smallest practical container (S. Zimicki, personal communication). All multidose presentations involve wastage; in 1993, the implementation team allowed for 10 % wastage (Pickering 1993). By contrast, the Afghanistan project uses 1-L bottles to avoid pouring from large into smaller containers; it was found that "the 1 litre bottles cost little or nothing more ... and are easier to account for when distributed (less subject to abuse)" (M. Rowland, personal communication).

Essential complementary supplies, such as measuring containers, bowls, plastic bags, indelible markers, and rubber gloves, must also be obtained. If the ITN project has provided them, they must be accounted for.

Most ITN programs and projects stress the importance of keeping registers of net purchasers and owners, who are potential clients for re-treatment services. Private-sector dipping services would also benefit from a record-keeping system that keeps track of when former clients' ITNs are due for re-treatment. A "tickler file," which automatically moves the eligible records to the front of the file, is good for this.

Training and Supervising Staff

In-service training

The need for refresher training about the malaria vector and its control should be assessed when reviewing knowledge and practices (especially prescribing) among health staff. Training sessions will be needed to introduce the staff to the ITN technology. Health professionals, as well as various community health workers and committee members (depending on implementation strategy), will need to be briefed on how activities will be organized, recorded, reported, supervised, and monitored. This briefing may be done, as it is in Kenya, by first training district teams, who are then responsible for running workshops at divisional level for village health committee members, community health workers, and traditional birth attendants. The relevant material is presented in the *Manual for the DHMT and Field Workers in Community-Based Malaria Control* (Hill 1992), which provides a practical model for preparing staff for an ITN program.

Interventions that aim to provide nets through local production will need to teach tailors and dressmakers how to assemble nets. I have seen examples of instructions for the Solomon Islands (S.R. Meek, personal communication) and for the community-based scheme in West Pokot, Kenya (J. Miesen, personal communication) (see also Figure 15).

Following a recipe

Just as the moment of administering vaccine to a child is the focal point of an immunization program, so the process of dipping the net is the focal point of an ITN intervention. Yet some instructions for preparing a solution of the correct strength are hard to understand. Researchers from The Gambia found that illiterate village health workers could not follow the calculations published by Schreck and Self (1985) and that the calculations took too long (Snow, Phillips et al. 1988). Publications from two established interventions contain gross errors in the quantities of water or insecticide to be added. The fact that highly trained professionals can make such mistakes emphasizes the importance of developing clear instructions that are easy to follow and result in an effective dose of insecticide on the net.

From an operational perspective, the best dip recipes lead users through the process step by step. The following is taken from the 2-week workshop in Sigoti, Kenya, in 1990, during which participants gave feedback on their first experience of preparing solution:

Due to hard calculation involved, the TOTs [trainers of trainers] promised to give a simple method of making a solution that can be used by the CHWs [community health workers] in the community. This involves use of ordinary containers available in the community — each CHW to bring any that takes the measurements from the measurement jar, and makes the mark against the container, takes note of the amount which must tally with the amount of water and finally the number of nets as per their sizes also taken into consideration.

How to prepare treatment solutions for different fabrics and the necessary safety precautions are explained in Chapter 2. The main problems of treatment in a PHC context are

❖ Calculating the correct amount of insecticide according to the chosen target dose and the size of the net; and

❖ Calculating the correct amount of water for diluting the insecticide, which is complicated by the fact that each type of fabric absorbs a different amount of water.

The recipes for the Solomon Islands offered 10 options: 5 categories of net (single Philippine, double Philippine, family Thai, single cotton, and double cotton) and 2 concentrations of permethrin (25% EC and 50% EC). From these options, the appropriate combination of water and insecticide must be chosen. For the Philippine and Thai nets, quantities of water and insecticide were given for 1, 5, 10, 20, and 50 nets (S.R. Meek, personal communication).

In Ecuador, the dipping is done by health promoters who must deal with a mixture of fabrics. Although 70% of nets were found to be cotton, the mother of the family frequently brought both synthetic and cotton nets to be dipped at the same time. A 15-m^2 synthetic net would absorb 1 L, whereas a 10-m^2 cotton net would absorb 1.4 L; recipes were prepared for each type of net (Kroeger and Alarçon 1993).

The variety of fabrics found in The Gambia may be greater than in any other ITN intervention. A recent user survey found that 60% of nets were nylon netting, 12% were nylon sheeting, 18% were light cotton and 9% were heavy cotton (S. Zimicki, personal communication). In 1992, the problem of differential absorbency was addressed by treating nets in succession, beginning with nylon nets, followed by light cotton and then heavy cotton nets (NIBP 1993a).

The complications introduced by changing any aspect of the insecticide were mentioned in the discussion on choosing insecticide. How can people's ability to follow a recipe be assessed if the recipe changes after the fieldworkers are taught to prepare the solution? The answer probably lies in setting clear guidelines on type of insecticide, dose, and formulation and ensuring that they are followed. If the private sector plays a larger role in net treatment, these issues must be resolved so that health staff and consumers can find out whether a private dipping service is safe and effective.

The only ITN implementation that sprays insecticide onto nets is in Sichuan Province, China; in other provinces, nets are dipped in bowls (Curtis et al. 1991). Spraying requires effective equipment and more personnel time per net, especially if households are scattered.

Providing the Service

Once the people responsible for mixing the treatment solution are adequately trained, many additional components are required to ensure that a treatment service is provided in a way that encourages net owners to use it.

Supplies other than nets and insecticide

The list of items that interventions have used includes measuring containers for insecticide and water, buckets for carrying water, large bowls or tubs in which to dip the nets, rubber gloves, indelible marker pens, plastic sheeting to collect solution that has dripped out of nets, and plastic bags for treating nets and carrying damp nets home. The list will vary according to the strategy chosen. What must the ITN program supply and what can households supply? For example, can the community provide buckets, bowls, and plastic bags, as in Ecuador? How many pairs of rubber gloves are needed per community, and how long do they last? Will community health workers supply containers to be marked up with the amount of insecticide to measure, as in Kenya (GOK–UNICEF 1990)? In The Gambia, a shortage of 5-L containers in the markets held up distribution in 1993 (NIBP 1993a) — this is the only mention of treatment activity hindered by supply shortage, but this is a topic that requires evaluation.

Availability and access to services

Two items — the net and the insecticide — must be provided at times and locations that are convenient for potential customers.

- ❖ *Bednets*: In Bagamoyo, purchasers found that with a single distribution point in the village, the process of distributing and treating nets took too long, so three separate distribution points were used in subsequent rounds (Makemba et al. 1995). In the Bamako Initiative projects, nets can be bought at any time from a community health worker, whose supply is kept at the community pharmacy (Hill 1991). These nets are illustrated in Figure 16.

- ❖ *Insecticide*: Treatment offered only in campaigns — twice per year, for example — must be scheduled for times when most net owners can reach the service.

Barriers to access include the limited time that insecticide is available in the village — some people find out about it only after it has been sent back (Pickering 1993) — and village health workers who refuse to dip dirty nets, even at the end of the session. Fees, both the amount and collection method, may also represent a barrier, especially if the household financial decision-maker is away. Other reasons why net owners may feel barred from access to the treatment service include their own

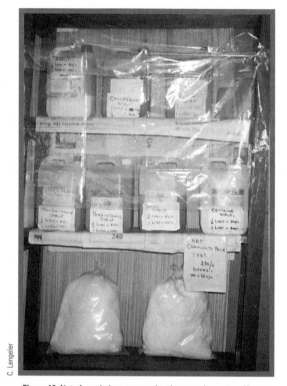

C. Lengeler

Figure 16. Nets for sale in a community pharmacy in western Kenya
(Bamako Initiative project).

own absence from the community when the service was offered, treatment offered at inconvenient times, social exclusion of sectors of the community, unwillingness or inability to reach the place where the service is offered, slow service or long waits for service, and the staff behaviour toward clients.

Barriers to access can be assessed by asking people why they did not get their net treated with insecticide. Two methodological features should be stressed:

❖ Such a survey must be done by independent interviewers — program staff should be interviewed as well, but neither they nor their colleagues from other communities can interview lost clients effectively; and

❖ The interviewers should record what people actually say, without editing, and should probe to get all factors — precoded categories conceal crucial nuances.

This approach has been used to great effect to evaluate immunization services; if done conscientiously, the responses from nonusers contain many pointers for improving the organization and accessibility of dipping sessions. In some cultures, people will not share dipping solution. If individual dipping is necessary, the details of operational planning (for example, choice of insecticide presentation and supplies of bowls) must take such preferences into account.

Washing the nets

Before treatment

Nets should be washed and dried before treatment. In areas where malaria is holoendemic and ITNs are in constant use or in locations where insecticide is available only at specific times, such as during a visit by a mobile team, ways must be found to tell people it is time to launder nets.

After treatment

With most interventions, users of ITNs are asked not to wash them for 6 months. Kenya's Bamako Initiative projects have more practical guidelines, suggesting that ITNs can be washed every 3 or 4 months, and advising fieldworkers to ask the local community health worker for re-treatment with permethrin (Hill 1992). This strategy is possible only if insecticide is stored locally. An operational decision to return insecticide to headquarters means that washed nets cannot be re-treated, and users are asked to adjust their washing of ITNs to fit the strategy. This arrangement may be unavoidable in isolated, rural settings with difficult access, as in Afghanistan, that are served by mobile teams. In such circumstances, coloured nets help users postpone washing them.

Will a strategy of treating nets on a 6-month cycle leave laundered ITNs with an inadequate dose of insecticide? The extent to which washing instructions are followed needs assessment. To improve access to services, especially after ITNs are washed, it may be necessary to explore strategies that adapt the application of insecticide to the laundering needs and preferences of net owners, as discussed in Chapter 2. Also in Chapter 2, the main safety issues are described, as are the variety of instructions for drying treated nets — out of direct sunlight, hung up, or laid flat on a plastic sheet or on bedding.

Monitoring, Supervision, and Evaluation

Monitoring, supervision, and evaluation are crucial to program management, but they are treated only briefly here because most aspects of general project management and evaluation apply also to ITN programs.

Choosing indicators

In field trials, most of the monitoring effort is directed toward measuring the effect of the intervention on malariometric, morbidity, mortality, and entomological parameters. This review discusses only the monitoring aspects required by nonresearch programs, and these are mostly process indicators. Financial monitoring has already been discussed.

Coverage is one of the most important parameters for monitoring, and different indicators are available: number of beds with nets, percentage of nets treated, percentage of the target group protected, and so on. Treated nets as a percentage of all nets was the measure of coverage used in The Gambia (NIBP 1993a). This has the great merit of being simple to estimate from registers of ownership and of net treatment. Villages with low coverage can be identified, and implementation problems can be followed up.

If a program chooses the number of households with at least one net as an indicator, this choice might help in monitoring equity, because it allows households with no nets to be identified. The percentage of households with at least one ITN would indicate program penetration. Some ITN programs have made certain target groups, such as pregnant women and children under 5 years of age, the highest priority and are designed to monitor coverage of these groups in particular.

At the outset, an ITN program may limit itself to monitoring relatively simple indicators, but as the implementation becomes more established, components of quality should be included, such as indicators of re-treatment (twice per year; immediately after laundering). However, a monitoring system that uses regularly reported data should not be burdened with every permutation and combination of variables. If a special investigation is needed, it should be done with sampling and surveys designed to answer specific questions arising from reported data and the observations of supervisors.

Operational indicators are essential for assessing the efficiency of service delivery and include the following:

❖ Availability of insecticide and nets;

❖ Stock-outs at point of delivery;

❖ Frequency of treatment services;

❖ Session size — how many people come with nets and how many nets are treated;

❖ Amount of insecticide used per session;

❖ Amount of solution discarded (wastage); and

❖ Amount of stock lost (leakage or theft).

These data indicate whether it is likely that the correct dose has been applied — for example, whether enough stock is used at treatment sessions to provide the target dose for the number of nets reported. To limit damage, any inconsistencies should be investigated immediately by supervisors and corrective action should be taken.

Another potential source of information on the quality of treatment is to ask consumers afterward whether the ITN killed mosquitoes and other nuisance insects. People's reports of "weak" insecticide led to the discovery of operational problems in The Gambia (U. d'Alessandro, personal communication).

Combined with indicators of coverage, information about session frequency and nets dipped per session will warn supervisors and managers of problems with the organization of services (for example, access and timing). Encouraging field staff to monitor participation by their clients will encourage a proactive approach.

The role of supervisors

The community has a role in monitoring and supervising fieldworkers, but field staff must also receive technical support from their trainers and supervisors. The most positive model is a perpetual feedback loop between training and supervision; if these tasks are done by the same people, they have no one to blame but themselves if skills are below standard.

It has been said that no ITN program will be sustainable unless the ministry of health or NGOs, or both, pay continuous attention to village committees. This attention can be in the form of evaluation, training and retraining, meetings, health education forums, and facilitating the exchange of ideas with other communities (Sexton 1993). The staff in these functions are the conduits of information from the field; during reviews of operational performance and strategies, these staff should be tapped for their invaluable experience.

Evaluation

Periodic evaluation serves the purpose of stepping back from daily detail and looking at implementation in a wider perspective. This process is usually strengthened when independent analysts are included in the evaluation team. The evaluation team can investigate queries about the program that are too complex to be answered from the regular reporting systems.

Apart from management problems, an evaluation can address equity and coverage of the target population by finding out who uses ITNs and who does not. A periodic evaluation can also gather information about the frequency with which people get them re-treated, how often they wash them, and whether they get them re-treated immediately after washing. This process would provide information for discussing how to make operational strategy compatible with good housekeeping.

Cost-effectiveness analysis

Few studies have assessed the cost effectiveness of ITN technology. Until the recent evaluation of the Gambian national program (Aikins 1995), this has always been done within field trials. Cost-effectiveness analysis, including analysis of the effects of operations management and the way a program is implemented, should produce important evidence of how the service can be organized and delivered more effectively. Such analyses should not be carried out until programs are sufficiently well established to provide several units (for example, districts or clinics) in the sampling design to permit assessment of variations in management performance.

Recommendations

The many areas needing further investigation and reporting have been highlighted throughout this review. A summary of specific recommendations is presented below.

❖ Operational research based on independent evaluations of past and current ITN programs would provide a useful body of information for planning the optimal choice of macro-level strategies, which would define various implementation models. Technical terms of reference should be developed, that specify the subjects that will be covered and include financing policies, accounting mechanisms, and economic sustainability of ITN schemes. The management roles of key staff should be included in the terms of reference. All sources of funding (household, community, government, NGO, or donor) should be included, and the issue of equity should be evaluated (for example, by comparing profiles of users and nonusers).

❖ Operational research is needed on the effects of some key issues at household level: the effect of the introduction of ITNs on the use and cost of other preventive measures; net-laundering practices, including the effect of small children in the household and of the net's colour; and the effect of different types of net on acceptability and uselife.

❖ Independent evaluations of fieldworkers' knowledge and practice of preparing solutions is urgently needed, including observation of fieldwork and analysis of stock records and net registers (sales and dips). Guidelines for net treatment should be modeled on successful interventions.

More general recommendations include the following:

❖ A clearing house for technical information should be established to supply updated and accessible technical material to anyone who asks. The technical authority of this service will depend on its independence from manufacturers and its use of feedback from ITN interventions. The EPI Unit of WHO might be a suitable model.

❖ Strategies for obtaining legal, administrative, and financial clearance, especially for imported insecticide, must be developed. It might be useful to consider experience with negotiating imports of vaccine and essential drugs.

❖ Donors providing large-scale support for vertical or integrated ITN programs should consider the short-term effects of the intervention on the existing net market.

❖ If the sustainability of an ITN program depends on continued support from outside the community, this support should be specified so that government agencies can make the necessary financial provision and establish systems for operating the program effectively.

Chapter 4

Promotion in Sub-Saharan Africa

S. Zimicki

Although nets are an old technology (Lindsay and Gibson 1988), surprisingly little is known about them in sub-Saharan Africa. Moreover, the notion of enhancing the protection they offer against malaria by treating them with insecticide has been considered for large-scale implementation only since the late 1980s (Curtis et al. 1991). Most information about the use of insecticide-treated nets (ITNs) in sub-Saharan Africa has been collected from efficacy trials designed to determine the effect of ITNs on malaria mortality and morbidity. Because efficacy comparisons involve "best-case" situations, these trials generally sought 100% coverage, usually by distributing nets free of charge and offering free insecticide treatment, as well as by intensive interpersonal promotion.

As countries consider incorporating ITNs into national malaria control programs, the question is how to achieve high, sustainable levels of appropriate use among those most at risk. National and regional programs cannot replicate the conditions of the efficacy trials. Thus, at least some people must bear some of the cost of nets and insecticide. In addition, many people are new to ITN use, and they need information about hanging nets, laundering them, and treating them with insecticide. Persuading people to buy nets and insecticide and informing them about using and re-treating ITNs will require special public-health communication efforts.

The public-health communication approach to improving health through changes in individual behaviour has been developed through experience and research over the past 50 years. The framework underlying public-health communication synthesizes "social marketing models of perception and perceived needs of the targeted audience, health education models of the components of behavioral intentions that influence willingness to act, and mass communication theories of the influences on transmission of messages from the source to the target audience" (NIH–NCI 1989).

Approaches to public health communication are characterized by the degree to which they emphasize these contributing elements. For example, the PRECEDE approach (Green et al. 1980) draws its name from its focus on the predisposing, reinforcing, and enabling factors that affect individual behaviour. The distinguishing characteristic of the social marketing approach (Walsh et al. 1993) is its use of audience, product, and channel analysis to develop marketing strategies for products as diverse as condoms and cancer screening. Although advocates of different approaches differ ideologically, the essential elements of the techniques used overlap substantially. All these approaches share not only the objective of improving health through behaviour change but also a requirement that design of the promotion should be based on situation analysis — that is, consideration of a limited number of elements, of which the most important are the health problem, its context, and the behaviour change(s) that would resolve it. This analysis leads to choices concerning the audience, the messages, and the channels to be used.

A brief review of each of these elements is followed by a description of how they were combined in three projects in Africa. There follows a general discussion of sociocultural elements related to using ITNs and other control measures to prevent malaria and nuisance biting. The next section briefly discusses the central problem of affordability, followed by reviews of essential information obtained from previous work on ITN interventions in sub-Saharan Africa. The final section presents a conclusion and some recommendations about promoting ITNs in sub-Saharan Africa and makes recommendations for research. In this review, insecticide-treated curtains are not mentioned specifically, but they can be promoted like nets.

Elements of Public-Health Communication

Effective public-health communication must consider who must be informed or persuaded, how to reach them, and what information to convey or arguments to make. These issues are, in turn, affected by assessments of the strongest motivations for the desired behaviour and the obstacles to its adoption, as well as the perceived characteristics of the "product" to be promoted. The audience, channels, and messages must all be considered in relation to each other and to the promotional objective.

Behaviour and product

The central considerations for developing public-health communication programs are examining the behaviour and its context and identifying the supports for the behaviour and the obstacles to change. Promotion has three pathways to behaviour change.

The first pathway is information. People may lack substantive information; they may not know that something is possible (measles can be prevented, there are ways to space children), that their behaviour increases their risk of disease (smoking causes lung cancer, mosquitoes carry malaria), or that they can benefit from changing their behaviour (frequent breastfeeding ensures a good supply of milk). Finally, they may need logistical information (when and where free vaccinations are given, where to obtain oral rehydration solution (ORS)).

The second pathway is skill. Learning new skills helps people achieve health goals. One example of this is the "pinch and scoop" method taught in Bangladesh for measuring salt and sugar for oral rehydration solution; another is the new emphasis on teaching women negotiation skills so they can persuade sexual partners to use condoms.

The third pathway is attitude change. Inculcating new standards for health or behaviour (a small family is a sign of wise behaviour, rather than shameful infertility) helps people set goals that differ from those set by their predecessors. A useful tool for selecting the specific behaviour to be promoted is the Behaviour Analysis Scale (Box 8).

Social marketers advocate explicitly defining the product being promoted. The product may be tangible, such as condoms, or intangible, such as the sense of being a good parent or responsible spouse. Tangible or intangible, it is useful to consider the product's attributes, such as price, perceived quality, and value to the audience, which may relate more directly to its image or "aura" than to its substance. For example, Coca Cola™ is preferred, not only for its flavour but also because it represents a lifestyle to which people aspire.

At the Dar es Salaam workshop, participants heard about the social marketing of condoms in Kenya and agreed that ITNs might also be promoted through social marketing.

Box 8

The Behaviour Analysis Scale

The Behaviour Analysis Scale rates behaviours on the following nine factors:

❖ Their potential impact on the identified health problem;

❖ Whether their positive consequences are immediate and apparent (potential for reinforcement);

❖ Their acceptability (compatibility with societal norms);

❖ How frequently people must perform them to achieve positive results;

❖ How consistently people must perform them to achieve positive results;

❖ The direct and indirect costs of performing them;

❖ Their similarity to other current behaviours;

❖ Their simplicity (the ease with which people can learn and undertake them);

❖ Whether they can be observed by others, which indicates whether social pressure can support performance (Graeff et al. 1993).

Considering the different aspects of the behaviour and, where relevant, of the product will aid in selecting the specific objectives of the promotion. This central choice in turn affects subsidiary decisions about audience, messages, and information channels.

Audience

Successful public-health communication addresses the needs (for information, skills, or reinforcement) of the primary audience, that is, the people who must act if the health objectives are to be achieved. Thus, mothers of small children are usually the main audience for promotions of homemade oral rehydration solution or breastfeeding. Some programs also identify secondary audiences, such as older women and husbands, because they influence mothers' decisions. Other potential secondary audiences are health workers, if contact with them to obtain information, supplies, or services is part of the desired behaviour, or shopkeepers, who might be a source of supplies and information.

For cost efficiency or equity, a public-health communication program may identify a segment of the population that must be reached; for example, rural people. This selection is especially useful when different information or distribution channels are suitable for different subgroups or when one subgroup needs particular information or skills.

Messages

Message content should relate directly to the audience's need for information, skills, or reinforcement of positive attitudes. Further, messages should be relevant, comprehensible, and easy to remember. Many failures in public-health communication can be traced to irrelevance in messages that arises from inadequate consideration of the perceptions of the audience. For example, planners sometimes believe that people are not doing something because they don't know about it and, therefore, "just have to be informed." However, for most preventive-health measures, such as exercising and giving up smoking, almost all research indicates that many more people know what they should do than actually do it. The deterrent may be the cost or difficulty of the behaviour or dislike of some of its perceived consequences.

In addition, sometimes message content directly contravenes "common-sense" knowledge. For example, one difficulty in promoting exclusive breastfeeding is the belief that everyone needs water, especially in hot weather, so both pediatricians and mothers are troubled by the idea of not giving young babies water, despite the growing number of studies demonstrating that breast milk alone is sufficient (J. Martines, personal communication).

Even when message content is relevant, it may not be comprehensible. Two main factors affect comprehensibility: the language used and the congruence of the message with established beliefs and attitudes. Messages must be in the language or dialect of the target audience, and the terms used must be used by that audience. Because local illness classifications frequently differ from biomedical classifications, several local terms may be needed to refer to one biomedical category. Similarly, for visual materials, in most cases, pictures of people are most useful if the audience can see the people in the picture as themselves. Whether this is more easily accomplished by using photographs or line drawings depends on the local situation. If the local preference is unknown, it should be ascertained during the early stages of pretesting.

If a message is not presented in a way that is consistent with accepted beliefs and attitudes, then it probably will not be believed. For example, cultures in which women are customarily veiled outside the home do not usually accept pictures of unveiled women, even if the depicted scene is at home, where women would ordinarily not be veiled. Ensuring that messages are comprehensible improves recall, as does simplicity. Ideally, people who are exposed to messages should remember them. If messages are too complicated, however, parts of them will probably be forgotten. Because messages to which people pay attention are more likely to be recalled, one approach is to present a "slice of life" situation that will catch their interest; for example, a mother with a sick child receiving advice about what to do. An additional advantage of dramatic messages is that people are more likely to listen and discuss what they have seen or heard with others. This secondary effect reinforces the message and stimulates the interest of those who have not yet been exposed to it.

A final characteristic of messages that relates to both relevance and recall is their specificity. Messages that tell people why or how to do something, such as "protect your child from measles, get him vaccinated for free at the health centre," are more likely to induce behaviour change than general ones, such as "breastfeeding is good for your baby."

Information channels

The correct choice of information channels — the media through which messages are transmitted — depends on relative impact and cost and hence cost effectiveness. Impact is a function of the proportion of the target audience reached by the channel, the frequency with which the audience can be exposed to messages, the channel's credibility, and the quality of the "spot" production. Costs to be considered are those of producing messages, of training people to deliver them, and of the actual delivery.

Interpersonal contact

Interpersonal contact is the channel with greatest impact. However, it is also the most difficult to manage on a large scale because the relatively low number of people any individual can reach implies either a large number of trained individuals or a long timeframe. Thus, interpersonal communication can be costly, because it can involve almost continuous training of new personnel to replace staff lost through attrition (volunteer programs commonly lose up to 30% of their workers in the first year after training), as well as recurrent training of all staff to maintain the consistency of the message.

Local media

Local media include drama groups, town criers, praise singers (griots), popular singers, and public announcements, such as by religious and political leaders at assemblies. The potential of local media is restricted by the possibly limited exposure of audiences to them, so they can be used to convey only simple, easily understood messages. Even dramas are susceptible to this limitation, as all aspects of the message must be conveyed in a relatively short period, and other elements of the drama (plot, characters, action) distract the audience.

Mass media

Increasing proportions of the population have access to mass media, primarily radio and television but also cassettes, videos, and films. Surveys in selected African countries indicate fairly high radio ownership, ranging from 62% to 83% in cities and from 30% to 66% in the rural areas (Table 14). In several countries, listenership is higher than ownership, indicating that people listen to friends' or relatives' radios. Overall listenership ranges from a low of 22% in rural Zimbabwe to a high of 89% in urban Namibia. Exposure to television is much lower and is confined mainly to cities.

A study of exposure to mass media in two villages in Ibarapa, western Oyo State, Nigeria, found that 75% of people listened to the radio (40% every day), 48% watched television, 29% read newspapers, and 19% read magazines (Brieger 1990). Fewer women than men listened to the radio; 34% of women said that they listened daily, compared with 46% of men. Further, 37% of women but only 14% of men said that they never

Table 14. Ownership and listenership (%) of radio and television (TV) in rural and urban areas of Africa.

Country	Radio: own		Radio: listen		TV: own		TV: listen	
	Urban	Rural	Urban	Rural	Urban	Rural	Urban	Rural
Lesotho	83.3	65.6	88.7	76.6	—	—	—	—
Cameroon	76.8	53.4	60.3	33.3	41.5	6.1	57.9	16.7
Namibia	80.3	66.2	88.9	75.2	46.0	2.7	55.2	6.3
Nigeria	81.8	48.6	82.1	43.8	57.1	7.8	67.4	11.7
Tanzania	62.5	29.8	76.6	36.3	3.4	0.1	9.5	1.4
Zambia	64.1	28.6	76.9	35.6	21.3	1.1	38.6	3.5
Zimbabwe	74.9	31.2	69.5	22.4	39.3	2.4	39.2	83.8

Source: HealthCom (Lesotho); Demographic Health Surveys.

listened. When listening was correlated with education, it was found that those with little or no education had both a lower frequency of daily listening (27%) and a higher proportion of never listening (38%) than those who had some education (daily, 55%; never, 13%). The main reason given for not listening was inability to afford a radio (mentioned by 68% of non-listeners).

Brieger concluded that radio would be useful for disseminating health information but should not be the only channel used because those for whom health programs are most relevant — women and low-income families — are least likely to be reached.

The major advantages of mass media are the consistency of the message and the potentially high frequency of exposure. It is also relatively easy to prepare radio messages in several languages. Although preparing radio spots can be expensive, radio is very cost effective. Radio and television dramas are used successfully to promote contraception for child spacing. Although dramas are technically complex, their format allows messages to be repeated over a long period; people get interested in the story, so the frequency of exposure to messages remains high.

Print materials

Print is a less expensive channel, but its reach is limited by illiteracy, poverty (newspapers and magazines cost money), and isolation — posters must be displayed where people will see them often. Leaflets are useful for complicated messages, such as mixing instructions, because they can be given away for people to keep for reference. Other useful print materials are calendars, which remind people of things that occur at specific times, and newsletters, which are particularly good for disseminating complex information among people with a common interest, such as volunteer workers.

Major constraints to extensive use of print materials in many countries are the wide variety of languages, some of them with no written form, and high illiteracy rates, especially among women. Demographic and health surveys carried out in 21 sub-Saharan countries between 1986 and 1993 showed that in only 7 countries had more than 80% of women in the 20–24 age group ever attended school (Carr and Way 1994). In the 12 countries where information was obtained about the proportion of children aged 6–15 attending school, the median for girls was 52%; for boys, 56%. Therefore, the visual components of print materials are particularly important and must also be assessed for comprehension and carefully tested (Haaland 1984; McBean 1989).

Summary

Reviews of large-scale health communication programs frequently conclude that decisions about the specific behaviour to be promoted, the approach to be taken, the target audience, the media channels to be used, and the messages to be sent must be based on information about the people and communities to be addressed (Hornik 1988; Robey et al. 1994). This formative research (also called planning research) should investigate the audience's perception of the problem, identify what the audience sees as the positive consequences of the behaviour (both immediate and long term), and ascertain the obstacles to adopting it. The research should also identify the language and terms that people use, as well as conventions that could affect visual materials.

A second important type of research is testing the message to learn whether the target audience will understand it and find it relevant. Several rounds of message preparation, testing, and revision are usually necessary.

In developing the final strategy for a program to promote a health behaviour, it is important to ensure that all the elements fit together. For example, even if most people listen to radio, promotion of a behaviour that requires complex new skills should not rely on radio messages alone; complex skills are much more effectively transmitted by interpersonal contact.

Three projects to promote oral rehydration solution in The Gambia, Swaziland, and Kenya are briefly described to illustrate how decisions about the elements of the promotion should be based on local information and how various elements should be combined in integrated strategies.

Three Examples of Health Promotion in Africa

Since the early 1980s, WHO has recommended ORS for treating diarrhea, particularly in infants and children. At first, "complete" solutions made with a prepackaged sugar, salt, potassium, and bicarbonate mixture were recommended, but it soon became apparent that many people could not get the packets and that it would be prohibitively expensive to supply enough packets for all episodes of diarrhea. Therefore, WHO began to recommend a simple, homemade solution of water, sugar, and salt in fixed proportions. Because high concentrations of either sugar or salt can be harmful and low concentrations are less effective, correct mixing is important. Both the Gambian and Swazi campaigns concentrated on teaching people the correct formula. The central issue in Kenya was to see whether ORS could be supplied commercially, but an important consideration in the evaluation was maintaining the quality of mixing when distribution of the packets moved outside the health system.

Example 1: Water–sugar–salt solution in The Gambia

Perhaps the most fully evaluated social-marketing project in sub-Saharan Africa has been the The Gambia Mass Media for Infant Health Project, carried out from 1981 to 1984 by the Ministry of Health, Labour, and Social Welfare, with the assistance of the Academy for Educational Development, and evaluated by Stanford University and Applied Communication Technology (Foote 1985). The project was designed to improve prevention and treatment of diarrhea in rural The Gambia. It approached its target audience, mothers of young children, through a combination of inexpensive radio spots and more expensive print materials and interpersonal contact by health workers and specially trained village volunteers. The project included 4 months of planning research using a variety of qualitative and quantitative techniques to find out about beliefs and practices concerning diarrhea, media use and habits, distribution systems for information and materials, and networks of local leaders to handle interpersonal communication.

A review of the developmental research (Rasmuson et al. 1988) revealed six circumstances that may account for the absence of a desirable behaviour:

❖ Lack of knowledge or skills;

❖ Incorrect or missing information about when to practice the behaviour;

❖ Lack of materials;

❖ Lack of apparent positive consequences of the behaviour;

❖ Positive consequences for engaging in incompatible behaviour; and

❖ Negative consequences that discourage the desired behaviour.

The objectives of the first year's campaign were then defined as informing mothers about the dangers of dehydration; how to identify "dryness" (dehydration); how to make a rehydration solution from water, sugar, and salt (WSS); how to feed a child with diarrhea; and when to take a child to the clinic. A series of radio messages presented during the first year of the campaign focused on dryness as the central danger associated with diarrhea. It told mothers that the symptoms of dryness are loss of weight, sunken eyes, dry skin, weakness, and listlessness and that they should immediately bring a child with these symptoms to the clinic. It emphasized the need to prevent dryness and explained how to make a medicine of WSS to prevent it. Complementary training materials for health workers and leaflets and posters on mixing WSS solution were also developed.

The campaign plan called for shifting emphasis according to the season and program phase. For example, in the first phase, carried out before the rainy season when most diarrhea occurs, messages focused on diarrhea and dehydration and its signs and introduced the idea of a "diet for diarrhea." At the same time, rural health workers were trained to mix and administer WSS, and they in turn trained 840 village volunteers. In the second phase, which took place during the rainy season, messages focused on mixing and administering WSS solution. Correct mixing was seen as the most difficult new behaviour, and some women testing the information materials had difficulty understanding the drawing indicating the amounts of WSS.

Therefore, to encourage mothers to ask health workers and volunteers for information and learn the mixing formula, a "happy baby" lottery was held (Elder et al. 1987). The leaflet of mixing instructions was a ticket. Each week for 4 weeks, 18 villages were randomly selected as lottery villages. In each village, the names of 20 mothers with mixing leaflets were randomly drawn, and the women were asked to demonstrate their mixing skills. Every woman who mixed WSS correctly received the 1-L drinking mug depicted on the mixing leaflet as a prize. Women who could also give correct answers to three of five questions about administering the solution to a child with diarrhea won a bar of soap and became eligible for the grand prize drawing, in which one woman from each of the five villages who had participated most actively in the contests won a radio-cassette recorder.

The evaluation revealed a high rate of exposure to the selected channels: 67% of 773 women interviewed in the four targeted divisions reported that they listened to radio daily or several times a week. With regard to interpersonal contacts, 80% of mothers of young children reported that they had visited a health centre in the previous 3 months, and most who lived in villages or towns with volunteers knew about them. These results indicated that appropriate media had been chosen.

Evaluation results also indicated high message awareness; for example, the proportion of women who knew how to mix WSS correctly increased steadily the first year and leveled at around 70% during the second year, when messages focused on feeding and sanitation. All health workers knew the correct formula. However, the campaign could not convince mothers that WSS would not stop diarrhea, probably because this fact conflicted with their belief that "medicine" recommended for diarrhea must stop it. The largest behaviour changes were seen in the use of WSS for home treatment of diarrhea. Over the course of 12 evaluation rounds held over 2 years (samples ranged from 885 to 1 041 women per round, varying because diarrhea is seasonal), the proportion of episodes treated with WSS increased from 4% to about 50%. Among cases treated only at home, the proportion treated with WSS rose from 22% to 94%.

Unfortunately, the success of this project was not institutionalized. A follow-up study of about 500 women carried out in 1987 indicated that 87% of women still knew about WSS, but that only 23% of them knew the correct proportions for all ingredients, compared with 78% in the last round of the previous evaluation (McDivitt and Myers 1987). Other research has demonstrated that people forget oral rehydration formulas unless periodically reminded (Chowdhury et al. 1988). At least part of this fall-off in knowledge and behaviour can also be attributed to the influence of health workers. Of the 101 women who brought children to clinics for the last episode of diarrhea, 63% reported that the health worker recommended some tablets, but only 18% reported that WSS was recommended and 21% reported that ORS packets were recommended (McDivitt and Meyers 1987).

Example 2: Sugar–salt solution in Swaziland

Another diarrhea-control campaign was carried out in Swaziland in 1984–85. This collaboration between the Ministry of Health, the Combatting Childhood Communicable Disease project, and the Mass Media and Health Practices program was evaluated by the Annenberg School for Communication (Hornik et al. 1986).

During the 5-month preparation phase, materials from The Gambia were assessed and adapted to Swazi conditions, and several investigations were carried out, including small anthropologic studies about beliefs and practices concerning diarrhea, a radio listenership survey, a review of ORS packet distribution practices, an analysis of current sugar–salt solution (SSS) formulas (three separate formulas had been taught in the past), a survey of mothers' practices in treating diarrhea, and a clinical study of potassium depletion, which had been identified as a particular problem in Swazi children with diarrhea.

A major decision based on results of the planning research, which indicated bottlenecks in the packet distribution system, was to focus on homemade SSS rather than packets. Because SSS would not address the problem of potassium depletion, the campaign strategy was modified to include instructions for mothers to begin SSS treatment at home, then to go to clinics, where potassium depletion could be treated. The recommended diet for children with diarrhea was also modified to include potassium-rich foods.

Radio materials (20 fifteen-minute dramas, 46 five-minute radio inserts, and 22 spot announcements) were prepared during a 10-week workshop on message development and radio production. Messages were based on results of the preliminary research. For example, because the formative research had indicated that one problem would be connecting dehydration with diarrhea, messages explaining the need for rehydration drew on local beliefs about the need to maintain a balance of fluids in the body.

As in The Gambia, the integrated campaign included radio broadcasts; print materials, including a leaflet about mixing and posters for clinics; and training workshops for health staff, extension staff, and local volunteers. However, the training workshops covered only about one-third of the country during the early part of the campaign. The short, 6-month campaign focused on using SSS mixed according to a new formula, maintaining feeding during diarrhea, and giving special feedings afterward.

Exposure to the campaign was high: about 85% of the 450 women interviewed during the evaluation were exposed to at least one campaign medium. Sixty percent of these mothers recognized the mixing leaflets, although only 20% could show one to the interviewer; 22% had visited clinics for a child's diarrhea during the campaign; 16% had contacted a local volunteer; and 62% reported listening regularly to at least two radio shows that broadcast campaign messages.

Knowledge based on the campaign messages increased substantially. For example, knowledge of the new SSS formula increased from 8% of 450 women interviewed just before the campaign to 26% of the 450 interviewed afterward. Evidence suggests that improvement may have been impeded by confusion about the different formulas. Knowledge of the correct amounts of water and sugar, which were the same in both the old and the new formulas, improved from 28% to 59%.

Reported use of SSS at home increased from 36% to 48% for episodes occurring in the month before the interview. Monthly information obtained from 23 of the largest health clinics in Swaziland indicated that among children coming to the clinic with diarrhea, previous use of SSS at home increased from 43% of those seen in September to 60% of those seen from November to April. Success was constrained by the incomplete implementation of the training portion of the strategy, the short duration of the campaign, and the complex baseline situation with three different formulas.

Example 3: Oral rehydration solution in Kenya

In contrast to the promotion of homemade solutions in The Gambia and Swaziland, the project in Kakamega District, Kenya, promoted packets of flavoured ORS available from commercial outlets in an area where unflavoured ORS was available free from PHC facilities (Kenya et al. 1990). The study was carried out in two divisions of Kakamega District; the flavoured packets were available and promoted in one division, and the other was maintained as a control.

A preliminary survey of 500 mothers investigated knowledge and attitudes about diarrhea and dehydration. It determined preferences for ORS flavours and indicated that 250-mL tin mugs were available in about 75% of households. In addition, a survey of 50 shopkeepers in the intervention area established their interest in adding ORS as an over-the-counter medicine.

Promotional materials produced in the local language included posters, billboards, and package leaflets, as well as a film. Pictorial instructions for mixing the solution featured a tin mug as the recommended measure for water. Shopkeepers were taught to show caregivers how to mix solutions; they were also asked to inform customers about free sachets available from clinics. The film, which was shown to mothers and children in the experimental division, promoted both the unflavoured sachets available at clinics and the flavoured sachets available in shops. Incentives for shopkeepers were a "reasonable margin" of profit (not specified); a system of volume discounts; and a requirement that they purchase the packets from the wholesaler in cash, which motivated them to sell the stock. A retail price of 5 Kenyan shillings[2] for four 250-mL sachets was chosen as both affordable and a bit more expensive than the cheapest over-the-counter medicines, to convince consumers that they were buying a reliable product.

Evaluation was based on the results of three surveys of 500 mothers carried out about 6 months apart in both areas. Exposure to the film was low; only 14% of respondents reported seeing it. The surveys did not include questions on how people learned about the commercial packets, but the researchers speculated that print materials were the most likely source of information.

Knowledge about ORS increased from 10% to 39% in the control area and from 20% to 55% in the experimental area. Ever use of ORS increased in both divisions, but more in the experimental division (from 18% to 54%) than in the control division (from 9% to 37%). Not only did more people in the experimental area use ORS, but they used about 0.5 L more per episode than people in the control community. Solutions obtained from 269 mothers in the experimental area and 252 mothers in the control area indicated that the accuracy of mixing the solution was about the same, with 31% in the experimental area and 35% in the control area preparing dilute solutions; 56% and 54%, acceptable solutions; and 13% and 11%, concentrated solutions.

What are the essential lessons?

Although all three projects had the same central objective — increasing the proportion of children with diarrhea who received appropriate treatment — strategies were adapted to local circumstances. Each project involved developmental research to identify those circumstances so that the campaign would target the correct behavioral objective.

In all three cases, the primary audience was people who would give solution to children. In the The Gambia and Swaziland projects, health workers and volunteers were not only important sources of information,

---

[2] In July 1996, 58.4 Kenyan shillings = 1 US dollar.

they were also secondary audiences for the radio spots and print materials. To ensure that people would have easy access to additional information, special attention was given to training both health workers and volunteers in The Gambia and Swaziland, although the Swazi effort was less successful. Shopkeepers in Kenya also received special training. In The Gambia, mothers were given an incentive to seek out people who had received special training, whereas in Swaziland and Kenya, trained people would be encountered mainly when children had diarrhea.

The Gambian and Swazi projects used radio, print materials, and interpersonal contact. The Kenya project used print materials (posters and billboards), package inserts, a touring film, and interpersonal contact. The film was a disappointment, which highlights the need to select media appropriate to the target audience and topic. Previously, a film had worked well to convey messages about agriculture to men, but the low proportion of women who reported seeing it in the 18 months of the project suggests that it was not a good choice for health messages about diarrhea (H.A. Mwenesi, personal communication).

In each project, the messages developed were specific and focused on the essentials: what the rehydration solution is for; when to use it; how to make it and administer it; where to get information, help, or packets; and how to feed children with diarrhea. Each project included all the elements for a successful promotion campaign (Box 9).

Most important, each project took account of the social aspects of human behaviour, which is rightly called "the forgotten factor" in the transmission of tropical disease (Gillett 1985). Indeed, a search in the literature using "bednet" and "behaviour" as key words produced far more citations about mosquitoes than about humans. Recent reviews of community participation in programs to control vector-borne disease (Winch et al. 1992; Service 1993) suggested that this inattention has contributed to the overall lack of success. If ITNs are to be promoted successfully, we need to understand their use better.

Sociocultural Aspects of ITN Use

Information needs

In planning the promotion of ITNs, the most important behaviours must be considered in relation to each essential element of public-health communication (objectives, product, audience, messages, and communication

Box 9

Elements for a successful promotion campaign

A successful promotion campaign incorporates the following four elements:

❖ Carefully chosen objectives based on consideration of local circumstances;

❖ Defined primary and secondary audiences;

❖ Channels selected for their suitability to the target audience; and

❖ A limited number of specific messages.

channels). Using ITNs to reduce malaria morbidity and mortality involves three main sets of behaviours:

❖ Acquiring ITNs;

❖ Using ITNs correctly and regularly; and

❖ Maintaining effectiveness with regular insecticide treatments.

Table 15 summarizes information required for planning promotional activities for each communication element and for the three behaviour sets outlined above. This information is relevant whether the approach selected is public-sector health education, social marketing with commercial distribution and promotion, or something else. The discussion that follows focuses on the elements in Table 15, although the items are not presented in strict order.

To select objectives for the promotion effort, the first question to ask is: What do people currently do about mosquito control in general and mosquito nets in particular? Information about current net users might indicate unprotected segments of the population for whom a special promotional effort should be made. These issues are discussed later in this section. The product (nets and insecticide) and people's preferences are reviewed extensively in Chapters 2 and 3.

Information essential to message development includes the reasons why people should get ITNs (perceived positive and negative consequences) and social norms concerning the importance of malaria as a health problem.

Table 15. Information about sociocultural aspects of main behaviours (net acquisition, use, and re-treatment) that will be helpful in planning the essential elements of promotional activities.

	Getting nets	Using nets appropriately	Re-treating nets
Objectives	How new is the behaviour? What mosquito prevention measures are currently used? Are there subgroups of the population that need special attention?		
Product	Preferences about net size, shape, etc.? Best distribution outlets? Best seen as health or household commodity? How affordable are nets?	Preferences about hanging? Do nets fit within household/sleeping arrangements? Perceived "hotness"?	Perceived effects of insecticide on insects, animals, children. How frequently are nets washed? Preferences regarding insecticide (smell, colour, etc.)? How affordable is re-treatment?
Audience	Who decides about purchases? Who pays?	Who takes care of nets?	Who provides insecticide? Who treats nets? Who pays?
Message content			
Positive consequences	Valued short- and long-term effects? Relative importance of disease prevention and nuisance reduction? Pregnant women and children seen as more susceptible? Does a net improve social standing? Impact on other insects? See mosquitos being killed? Can reduction in disease be perceived?		
Negative consequences	Do only certain members of the household (males, senior members) get nets, use them, or get them treated?		
Obstacles	Affordability of nets? Seasonality of money supply, mosquito density, malaria transmission?		Affordability of insecticide?
Norms	Is malaria seen as a problem? What is relation between local and biomedical classification?		
Channels	Usual sources of information and advice for commodities? Frequency of contact with health centres, shops, markets?		Usual source of supplies? Who do potential customers see and respect?

These aspects are discussed in "Reasons for Acquiring and Treating Nets," pp. 132–136. The affordability of nets and insecticide, an important obstacle to the desired behaviour, is discussed in "Affordability," pp. 136–140. Finally, the available information on Communication Channels in ITN programs is discussed in "Communication Channels Used in ITN Programs," pp. 140–147.

Information sources

The information presented below has been summarized from several types of sources:

- ❖ Studies of recognition and treatment of malaria and measures to control nuisance insects;

- ❖ Published and unpublished reports of efficacy trials and implementation programs; and

- ❖ Interviews with selected researchers, implementors, and representatives of donor organizations.

Particular weight is given to experience from implementation programs detailed in Chapter 3.

Measures to prevent mosquito bites

A few surveys have reported on the most common measures against mosquito bites (Table 16). Surveys carried out in Yaoundé and Douala, Cameroon, revealed high proportions of households doing something to prevent mosquito bites (Desfontaine et al. 1989; Desfontaine et al. 1990). Large differences in the proportions of households using specific measures in the two towns reflect the lower prevalence of mosquitoes in Yaoundé (800 m above sea level) than in Douala. A nationally representative survey in Malawi (Ziba et al. 1994) indicated a much lower prevalence of preventive methods in poorer rural communities, although the researchers included questions about methods requiring no cash outlay, such as burning leaves and dung. Higher rates of coil and spray use and a similar rate of bednet use were identified in Uriri, a community outside Kisumu, Kenya (Sexton et al. 1990). In the two villages studied in that community, 38% of families had indoor cooking fires, considered a mosquito deterrent.

In Malawi, use of coils, bednets, and sprays was positively correlated with income, whereas use of nonpurchased methods was only weakly

Table 16. Use of different mosquito-prevention measures (%) in selected locations in Africa.

	Coils	Spray	Nets	Smoke	Any	Source
Yaoundé	18	60	15	—	84	Desfontaine et al. (1989)
Douala	37	40	48	—	91	Desfontaine et al. (1990)
Malawi	16	11	7	18	52	Ziba et al. (1994)
Uriri	56	40	9	38	—	Sexton et al. (1990)

negatively correlated with income. Expense was the reason given by 57 % of people who did not use coils and 76 % of people who did not use bednets (Chitsulo et al. 1992). Ettling et al. (1994) showed that very poor households were not only less frequent users of purchased methods but also, among households that used a method, spent less per year on it. This pattern also appears in western Kenya (J. Hill, personal communication).

Current use of nets

Although information about sub-Saharan Africa is relatively sparse, it is clear that there are great variations, not only in the proportion of households using nets in a given area but also in the proportion of use within households. Bednet use seems to be higher in West Africa, especially The Gambia, than in East Africa and higher in cities than in rural areas.

A nationwide survey of 360 compounds in rural areas of The Gambia, carried out during the high mosquito season of 1991, indicated high levels of net use: 58 % of the 3 867 beds enumerated had a net (d'Alessandro et al. 1994). Net use was higher in the central region (76 % of 1 293 beds enumerated, with more than 90 % of those used by pregnant women and young children) than in the eastern or western regions (about 51 % of the beds enumerated, with 55–65 % of those used by pregnant women and young children). Use was related to ethnicity, as it had been in earlier studies in the central region (Bradley et al. 1986; MacCormack and Snow 1986). However, a recent study indicates that most of the observed ethnic differences can be explained by factors predicting mosquito density (Thomson et al. 1994).

Aikins et al. (1993), who carried out earlier work in the central region, pointed out the difficulty of establishing children's sleeping habits. Young children usually sleep with their mother and are thus protected by her bednet (MacCormack and Snow 1986). Older children usually sleep with a parent, another adult relative, other siblings, or (rarely) on their own and may not have access to a net. Adolescent boys may sleep outdoors (Aikins et al. 1994) and are thus much less likely to have access to a net. The use rate among boys under 10 years of age was slightly (3–8 %) lower than that of adults; the use rate among girls was about the same as that of adults. The variation in results between this study and the national survey is probably attributable to a difference in age groupings.

Rates of net use approaching those reported from The Gambia were reported from a survey of 600 households in urban Brazzaville, Congo: 73% of households owned at least one net (Carme et al. 1992). A survey by the Danish International Development Agency also identified a high use rate (69%) in periurban Bandim, Guinea Bissau (Aikins et al. 1994).

Intermediate rates of net ownership have been reported for Douala, Cameroon, where 48% of the 420 households surveyed owned at least one net (Desfontaine et al. 1990), and in the Savalou region of Benin, where a survey of 181 households indicated that 41% used nets (Rashed et al., unpublished),[3] with higher net use by adults than by children.

A survey of 420 households in Yaoundé, Cameroon, indicated that nets were used in only 14.5% of households, although pregnant women and children were more likely to use them than others in the same household (Desfontaines et al. 1989). Anecdotal evidence indicates that few people (less than 10%) use nets in villages near Bo, Sierra Leone (Aikins et al. 1994), north of Ouagadougou in Burkina Faso (A. Habluetzel, personal communication), and in the Navrongo study area in northern Ghana (F.N. Binka, personal communication). In East Africa, very low rates of net use were found in Uriri, Kenya, and Malawi (Table 16). A baseline survey in western Kenya identified only 15% of households that owned at least one net (Hill 1990), and this rate was even lower in Kilifi, on the Kenyan coast (E.S. Some, personal communication), in Bagamoyo, on the Tanzanian coast (Makemba et al. 1995), and in southern Tanzania (C. Lengeler, personal communication). These low figures of current net use are probably representative of large areas of rural Africa.

Social and age differentials in net use

Despite low use rates overall, it appears that, in most places, at least a few people already use nets. In areas of low net use, the association with socioeconomic status may be strong. For example, in Malawi only 4–5% of 798 very poor households and 304 poor households own at least one net, whereas 10% of the 292 moderately wealthy and 19% of the 131 wealthy households do (Chitsulo et al. 1992).

In contrast, in high-use areas, socioeconomic status seems to have relatively little influence on use. In the central region of The Gambia,

---

[3] Rashed, S.F.; Johnson, H.; Dongier, P.; Gbaguidi, C.C.; Lalaye, S.; Capochichi, S.; Ménou, J.; Tchobo, S.; Gyorkos, T.W.; Joseph, L.; MacLean, J.D.; Moreau, R. Les attitudes, connaissances et pratiques vis à vis de la malaria et l'utilisation des moustiquaires dans le centre de la République du Bénin. (Submitted for publication.)

Aikins et al. (1993) found no correlation between use and education, occupation, or income, although ownership of radios and cassette players was significantly more frequent among net owners. In Brazzaville, Congo, ownership was weakly related to comprehension of French, which is associated with socioeconomic status (Carme et al. 1992).

Net use is likely to be higher in urban than in rural areas. It is also associated with education and wealth, suggesting that a net is a prestige item, one that people want to acquire. Consequently, ensuring that high-risk groups have adequate access to nets may be difficult. For example, the large-scale efficacy trial in Ghana originally intended to distribute nets only to high-risk groups but finally distributed nets to all family members because men complained of being left out and project staff feared that men would take nets issued for women and children (F.N. Binka, personal communication). This reaction probably reflects a widespread belief that such beneficial items should not go only to women and children but should either be shared by all household members or go to the senior men of the household.

Confirmation of this concern came also from the Bagamoyo project (Winch and Makemba 1993). After nets were sold, inquiries revealed that men used them most, followed by women, and then children. As children did not usually sleep with their mothers after the age of 2, they were least likely to be protected. This pattern, which differs from that seen in areas where net use is high, warrants concern because it indicates that groups at greatest risk may not benefit from net programs.

Reasons for Acquiring and Treating Nets

There are two main motivations for acquiring and using a net:

- ❖ Protection from malaria; and
- ❖ Protection from being bitten by mosquitoes and other nuisance insects.

Protection from malaria

Information from several surveys (Table 17) indicates little correlation between net use and the perceived role of mosquitoes in transmitting malaria (inferred from whether people mentioned mosquitoes when asked the cause of malaria).

Table 17. Knowledge about the cause of malaria and frequency of net use in selected locations of Africa.

Area	Say mosquitoes cause malaria (%)	Use nets (%)	Sample size	Source
Central Gambia	28	86	996	Aikins et al. (1993)
Ibarapa, Nigeria	28	0	1 935	Ramakrishna et al. (1990)
Malawi	55	7	1 531	Ziba et al. (1994)
Savalou, Benin	75	41	184	Rashed et al. (unpublished, see footnote 3)

Some of the variation in causal attribution is probably an artifact of questioning: if people are allowed only one response and the question concerning cause implies "What increases the likelihood that you will get malaria?" then responses such as "the rains" may be given even by those who believe in transmission by mosquitoes. Therefore, these surveys may underestimate comprehension of the link between mosquitoes and malaria.

Nevertheless, in some places people seem to be unaware of the link between mosquitoes and malaria. Agyepong (1992) described such an area in southern Ghana, where the biomedical and local causal models for malaria are completely dissimilar. The Adangbe people believe that *asra* — a local disease classification based on signs and symptoms, that includes malaria, as well as other diseases with similar signs and symptoms — is caused by prolonged exposure to excessive heat, either from the sun or from being too near a fire. People think that little can be done to prevent the disease, as it is impossible to avoid heat in an equatorial country such as Ghana. Agyepong warns that in this situation, malaria-control programs can expect, at best, passive compliance with control activities and that sustained control can be achieved only with constant inputs from outside. This assessment is undoubtedly true in the short term, but a question remains: Do people recognize a reduction in malaria as a consequence of an intervention?

Even in areas with less divergence between local and biomedical disease classifications, information about local disease classifications may be helpful in understanding why people use nets in some seasons but not in others. For example, a study in Bagamoyo indicated that the local term *homa* encompasses both mild and severe biomedical malaria (Winch et al. 1994). Various kinds of *homa* are recognized, and each type is thought to have a different cause. Although one mild type, *homa ya malaria*, is thought to be caused by mosquitoes, it is not coextensive with biomedically defined malaria. On the Kenyan coast, mild malaria is understood to be related to mosquitoes, but cerebral malaria, the severe form, is clearly identified as a spiritual disease for which any western biomedical treatment or prevention is ineffective (Mwenesi et al. 1995). Other local disease classifications can apply to episodes of malaria, depending on the circumstances under which people fall ill.

In general, in areas where local and biomedical classifications differ, people tend not to recognize episodes of malaria in seasons of low mosquito density as actually caused by mosquitoes. This lack of recognition affects their willingness to use nets.

Reduction of nuisance biting

Concern about ignorance of mosquitoes' function in malaria transmission has led to a suggestion that reducing nuisance biting should be emphasized as the reason to use ITNs. This suggestion is supported by the finding that reports of high indoor mosquito density is associated with net use in West Africa (Aikins et al. 1994). The same is also seen at national level in Burundi (van Bortel 1996) and The Gambia (Thomson et al. 1996). Nearly everyone uses a net in certain neighbourhoods in Douala, Cameroon, that are particularly suitable habitats for *Culex quinquefasciatus* (Desfontaine et al. 1990). In the Bagamoyo net project, people living in the centre of villages where *Culex* densities were higher were also more likely to use their nets (Winch and Makemba 1993).

People asked about ITN benefits usually talked far more about reduction of mosquito nuisance than about reduction of malaria. Reduction of nuisance biting is undeniably the more immediate, frequent, and perceived consequence of ITN use. However, avoiding nuisance seems insufficient as a motivation for year-round ITN use; nonuse seems fairly common, especially during the low mosquito season. For example, in the 1992 Malawi national survey, only about 66% of households with nets reported that they had been used the previous night (Chitsulo et al. 1992).

Several ITN trials included night visits to check use. In one efficacy trial in western Kenya, 85% of people with nets claimed to use them regularly, but night visits indicated a use rate of about 70–73% during the dry season. Nonusers said either that they had "forgotten" or that it was too hot for nets (Sexton et al. 1990). In the same area the next year, compliance was measured through unannounced night visits (from 9 to 11 PM) monthly for 3 months (Beach et al. 1993). The first compliance visits, at the end of the dry season, detected use rates of 78%. Visits during the following months showed higher use rates, varying from 86 to 98 %. The researchers attribute this improvement to increased mosquito densities and biting rates during the high-transmission season. A similar pattern of seasonal use was reported from the Kenyan coast (E.S. Some, personal communication).

Interestingly, Lindsay, Snow, Broomfield et al. (1989) noted less net use in villages where all nets were treated with permethrin. They attributed this to the perceived reduction in mosquito bites in houses with permethrin ITNs. This tendency for people to avoid using nets unless mosquitoes actually bother them is a problem that must be addressed because malaria transmission can occur when mosquito densities are low (Thompson et al. 1994).

Other ITN benefits

Another important benefit of ITNs, particularly when they have been laid on beds to dry, is their effect on other nuisance insects. The nets can eliminate bedbugs and headlice completely and reduce the number of other flying and crawling insects (Lindsay, Snow Armstrong et al. 1989). As reported from a trial in Tanzania (Njunwa et al. 1991):

> In the days after the bednets were distributed, villagers reported enthusiastically, and without prompting, on the death of mosquitoes near bednets and the disappearance of other pest insects, including bedbugs, fleas and even, in some cases, cockroaches.

Other ITN benefits include privacy, protection from dust and roof debris, and warmth during the cold season (MacCormack and Snow 1986; Aikins et al. 1994; Rashed et al., unpublished, see footnote 3).

Should disease reduction or nuisance reduction be emphasized?

Although nuisance reduction is the reason most frequently cited for ITN use, two problems arise when only this aspect is emphasized. First, it may not be enough to motivate people to spend money on nets or insecticide treatment when cash is short. If an ITN is seen only as a comfort, it may be ranked not only below food but also below other pleasures, such as tobacco. Second, if ITN use is seen only as a way to ensure a good night's sleep, adults, especially men, are most likely to get preference. People in some communities believe that children sleep more soundly than adults and are less bothered by mosquitoes.

In view of these possibilities, the wisdom of promoting ITNs to reduce nuisance biting must be carefully considered. In any case, some emphasis should also be given to protection from malaria. Local circumstances should determine whether local terms that overlap the biomedical classification of malaria can be used or whether a biomedical classification should be introduced. More information is still required on the perceived importance of the two sets of benefits and on whether the reasons for acquiring and using ITNs change over time.

Rumours

Popular rumours can seriously hinder a project. These rumours can be based on fact (for example, one person's experience of side effects) or be completely unfounded (for example, if one person or a group in the community sees the program as a threat). The need for good rapport with the community and local authorities is crucial both for preventing damaging rumours and for dealing with them as they arise. Therefore, a good overall communication strategy is essential.

Experiences reported by participants of the Dar es Salaam workshop suggested that caution should be exercised when designing programs that emphasize the idea of killing insects, as this idea might indue a fear of toxicity among parents of young children and a consequent rash of negative rumours.

Affordability

Evidence on affordability as a barrier to net use

The strong correlation between income and net ownership noted for low-use areas suggests that the cost of nets deters use. In all studies that elicited reasons for nonownership, the most frequent response was the expense of purchasing a net: 76% in Malawi (Chitsulo et al. 1992) and 58% in both Savalou, Benin (Rashed et al., unpublished, see footnote 3), and The Gambia (Aikins et al. 1994). In Brazzaville, Congo, Carme et al. (1992) noted an overall proportion of 49% of nonowners giving expense as the reason, ranging from 87% among poor people to 36% among wealthy people.

The major barrier to net acquisition reported by respondents during the first distribution period of the Bagamoyo project was lack of money when nets were sold (Bagamoyo Bed Net Project 1992). In most rural areas, cash availability is seasonal: people get money at harvest and often spend most of it by the beginning of the next planting season. Unfortunately, in areas with seasonal transmission, mosquito nuisance and malaria transmission are usually low during the period when cash is most available, and thus less immediate incentive exists to acquire a net at that time.

In an evaluation of a UNICEF-supported project in western Kenya, people were asked how many nets they thought they could afford to buy in a year at two different prices, 60 and 100 Kenyan shillings (Hill 1991). The consistency of the answers to the two questions suggested that people had a definite sum in mind that they thought they could spend on nets.

Another important factor in affordability, at least initially, is the number of nets a household needs. For example, in Tanzania, the number of nets required by each household was a major practical obstacle because people were reluctant to purchase only one net and leave other household members unprotected (J.N. Minjas, personal communication). The number of nets required will be affected not only by family size and sleeping patterns but also by the need to accommodate population movements. Travelers must either take a net with them, leaving their own household short, or risk being unprotected while away. Therefore, households need extra nets for travelers to take away and for visitors to use.

Problems in estimating affordability

When considering what people can afford, we cannot assume that money currently spent on preventive measures and malaria treatment is available for purchasing or treating an ITN because we cannot assume that ITNs will replace other measures, such as aerosol insecticide or coils. Aikins et al. (1993) reported that net users spent less on coils than nonusers ($0.90 per month, compared with about $1.20). However, ITN owners still sit outdoors when mosquitoes are biting and sleep outdoors in hot weather or before the harvest, when people sleep in the fields to protect crops from animals (Winch and Makemba 1993).

Several concerns must be addressed when considering expenditures on treating malaria and fever. First, ITN use does not prevent all episodes of malaria. Further, many illnesses treated as malaria are probably not in fact clinical malaria, so the amount of money released by malaria prevention can be overestimated. Finally, it is not clear that people consider potential saving on disease-related expenditure when deciding what to spend on prevention.

The issue of subsidies

One way to ease the problem of affordability is to subsidize nets and insecticide. Quite apart from the cost to the subsidizing institution or organization (see Chapter 3), two problems arise from special efforts to supply affordable nets:

- ❖ Possibility of resale; and
- ❖ Purchase by nontarget groups.

In Tanzania, 6 months after distribution, nets disappeared at rates of 6–34% in three villages; in a fourth village, the rate was 29% after 12 months (Njunwa et al. 1991). Up to 8% were reported stolen; the survey team did not find the other nets because they were hidden from thieves, lent to relatives, taken by someone who moved away, or surreptitiously sold. Except for nets hidden from thieves, all were unavailable to the families supposed to be using them.

In the Kilifi efficacy trial, in which nets were distributed free, 7–20% of the nets were not seen by survey teams on their rounds (E.S. Some, personal communication). The most frequently cited reasons for their disappearance were that they had been taken elsewhere (just over 50% of those not seen), that they had never been issued (16%), that they had been stolen (6.2%), or that they had been burned (4.6%).

In Benin, research is under way to determine who bought nets produced by the project. Project staff believe that in the project zone, more were bought by people from the local city than by rural people. It also seems clear that some nets are bought by urban people from outside the project zone, but the rate of this "leakage" is unknown (S.F. Rashed, personal communication).

The amount of leakage in any project is directly related to the price difference between project nets and commercial nets. If the project is based on full cost recovery or subsidies are small, leakage will be low. Setting project net prices close to commercial levels will discourage leakage and may increase the nets' perceived value. On the other hand, higher prices would reduce affordability.

Affordability of insecticide for re-treatment

Although most people are enthusiastic about the results of treating nets with insecticide when it is offered free, it is difficult to get them to re-treat nets when they are asked to pay even a modest amount.

The clearest example of this is in The Gambia, where dipping and payment for dipping were phased in so that several villages received free insecticide for several years before having to pay. Uptake rates were about 85% the first year that dipping was offered free, 75% during the second year, and then fell to 25% or less when people were asked to pay $0.5, about the price of a box of mosquito coils. This reluctance to pay for re-treatment was also seen in the Podor project in Senegal (M.C. Giancarlo, unpublished).[4] When payment was introduced ($0.80 for a cotton net and $0.40 for a nylon net) the proportion of people bringing nets for re-treatment dropped by two-thirds. Because the major reason seemed to be the cost of treatment, an experiment was carried out in three villages. In the first, when dipping was offered at $0.10 per net, coverage was 80%. In the second, when the full price was requested but a delayed payment option was offered, coverage was 75%. In the third village, when people were required to pay the full price at the time of dipping, only 40% coverage was achieved.

A 1994 survey in The Gambia asked respondents whether they had treated their nets in 1993, nearly a year before, and why they dipped or did not dip (Zimicki et al. 1994). About half cited lack of money: the cost of dipping all the household nets when cash was short was simply impossible. Virtually no one considered dipping some but not all their nets. Others, who seemed able to afford the insecticide, gave reasons suggesting that inconvenience or low priority were major factors: they were traveling, were not aware of when dipping was offered, or considered the dipping site too far away. Similar reasons were given in the Bagamoyo project, which also found that it was much more difficult than expected to convince people to bring nets for re-treatment (Winch and Makemba 1993). However, they pointed out that re-treatment was not emphasized in any of the promotions, which had instead focused on acquiring nets and using them correctly.

---

[4] M.C. Giancarlo. 1990. Rapport de mission. Projet FED "Programme d'appui au Développement de la région de Podor" — Volet Santé. Unpublished. 43 pp.

In The Gambia, questions were asked about "willingness to pay" for treatment under various hypothetical conditions (Zimicki et al. 1994). Almost 90% of people expressed interest in treating their nets for $0.50, but nearly one-third of these people qualified the answer with "if I have the money." Fewer than one-third of all users said they would pay $1.00, even for better insecticide. Although responses to hypothetical questions are notoriously bad predictors of actual behaviour, this response pattern suggests a high level of price sensitivity. Family-planning experience has shown that price is important to program success. In one project, an increase of $0.01 in the price of condoms resulted in a large decrease in coverage (Ciszewski and Harvey 1994). An analysis of coverage (sales per capita) against price relative to gross national product (GNP) for 24 condom programs showed a strong correlation between price and sales; in the most successful programs, the price of 100 condoms is less than 1% of per capita GNP (Harvey 1994).

Communication Channels Used in ITN Programs

Interpersonal contact

Because all efficacy trials conducted to date have been relatively small, they have involved intense interpersonal promotion. For example, at the beginning of the Kilifi project, 2 months were spent informing government officials, local community leaders, health officials, and the community (Snow 1994). Community education was done during preliminary village meetings, home visits for registration and net delivery, and group meetings with household representatives the day after net delivery. When nets were first distributed, project staff spent about half an hour in each household demonstrating how to hang and use them (Marsh 1994). Similar procedures were followed by other efficacy trials, but it is unlikely that large-scale programs could use paid staff for this kind of promotion.

One program in Zimbabwe relied almost exclusively on personal contact between clients and staff at a few clinics. This reliance seriously limited the number of sales and compromised the program (T. Freeman, personal communication). Even small programs need a certain volume of sales and therefore should opt for a more widespread promotion strategy. For example, in The Gambia, selected shopkeepers were given supplies of insecticide sachets on consignment, along with promotional and informative leaflets to distribute to buyers. This direct promotion was backed up by radio spots and other forms of communication.

Village health and bednet committees

One low-cost interpersonal promotion method is entrusting some program tasks to villagers. Village health committees are integral to the Bagamoyo bednet project, to the UNICEF-supported project in western Kenya, and to the Gambian national ITN program. In The Gambia and Kenya, village health workers have specific responsibilities related to the distribution of nets and insecticide, and their promotion (Figure 17). In Bagamoyo, Tanzania, net committees were formed in each village.

The Bagamoyo project has provided the best documentation of the difficulties associated with village committees (Makemba et al. 1995). Forming the committee was arduous enough: 20 villagers chosen at random, members of the village government, and project employees who worked in the village were each asked to nominate five people, and the five community members most frequently nominated were asked to form the committee. This process was time consuming because everyone asked for nominations wished to discuss the committee's responsibilities. Moreover, people tended to nominate village elders. Although

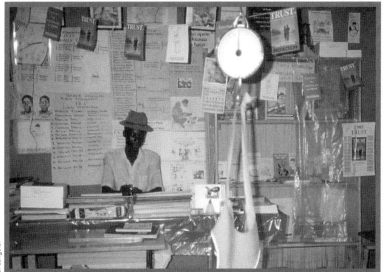

Figure 17. Community health worker in western Kenya: an important intermediary for health promotion.

elders were known and trusted, most had other responsibilities that precluded full involvement in committee activities, or they found the project too demanding.

Village committees seem difficult to maintain. In Bagamoyo, 11 of 13 health committees formed for another PHC project several years before the net project began had been dissolved. By the third year of the ITN project, some of the new village committees were suffering strong internal strains and were not expected to continue. An important lesson learned here was that special committees must keep on good terms with village governments. In the Bagamoyo project, members of village governments were invited to attend the day-long orientation seminar for the village committee members (Makemba et al. 1995). Village health and bednet committees also need good contacts with Ministry of Health staff (J. Hill, personal communication).

Theatre

The Burkina Faso and Kilifi efficacy trials and the Bagamoyo net project all used theatre groups to disseminate information. The Burkina Faso trial hired a professional group from Ouagadougou and worked with them to produce a play that toured the whole study area over 3 months, presenting 40 shows seen by people from 160 villages. The script covered the following ideas: malaria kills children, mosquitos are not only a nuisance but also disease vectors, and treated curtains protect children; the play also showed how to use treated curtains (A. Habluetzel, personal communication).

The Kilifi trial experimented with a play to teach upper-level primary-school pupils how to use ITNs, in the hope that they would bring the information home to their parents (Marsh 1994). One stimulus for the experiment was a home survey that highlighted three areas of particular difficulty: what to do with nets when traveling, how to position the bottom of a net, and how to wash nets.

This survey also indicated that parents would listen when their older children gave them new information. The drama incorporated eight messages:

- ❖ Reasons for using nets;

- ❖ Ownership and responsibility for nets;

- ❖ Importance of using nets every night of the year;

❖ Positioning the bottom of a net;

❖ Household responsibility for repairs and for reporting stolen or damaged nets;

❖ Importance of having the net stay when people travel, or having it move only with children under 5 who use it regularly;

❖ Importance of only washing nets just before treatment and necessity for re-treatment every 6 months; and

❖ Organization of the trial and distribution of nets to people in the control group after the trial.

After the performance, guided small group discussions reinforced these messages. Pupils were also assigned homework that required discussing ITNs with their parents.

An evaluation of the experiment indicated that the drama was successful as a source of information for the students. They understood and recalled all the information, except the need to use nets all year and the trial design. Recall of information about positioning the bottom of the net and about the re-treatment interval was somewhat weak. Results of the homework assignments indicated that pupils did talk with their parents about ITNs, but discussions with parents at later meetings indicated that the pupils were able to transmit less information to their (predominately male) parents than had been hoped. The final evaluation of this experiment, based on interviews carried out with mother's of 100 students, indicated that whereas most mothers were aware of the teaching program only about a third could recall any specific message (V. Marsh, personal communication).

During the first round of net distribution in Bagamoyo, a play presented on distribution day was intended to show how to use nets. However, it was inefficient as a source of information because not everyone saw it. This experience highlights the importance of considering exposure levels before selecting media.

Print materials

Projects have used several kinds of print materials. The Kilifi project produced flip charts to be used during home visits (Snow 1994), and the Bagamoyo project produced posters and booklets for net users and village committee members (Bagamoyo Bed Net Project 1992). The Gambian national net program developed one-page leaflets for distribution in PHC villages and through shops selling insecticide (Greenwood 1994). A sample of the art is shown in Figure 18.

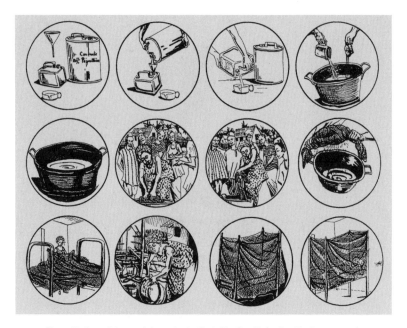

Figure 18. Artwork from an information leaflet in The Gambia (national bednet program).

Some projects hold drawing competitions to involve children in learning more about nets and malaria. The resulting artwork may sometimes be used in project print materials. Figure 19 shows an example of such artwork. Drawn by 18-year-old Abrahami Majitanga, the figure depicts *matumizi ya chandarua* ("correct use of the net") and *dawa yake inauwa wadudu* ("the treatment kills insects"). The competition was sponsored by the Rotary Net Project at the Ifakara Centre (Kilombero District, Tanzania).

All drawings, whether produced in a student contest or by an artist, must be pretested with the audience that will be using the project materials. The extensive development and testing process used in the Kilifi project and the more abbreviated process used in The Gambia indicated several problems likely to be encountered when producing visual materials for other areas (V. Marsh, personal communication; K. Cham and S. Zimicki, personal communication). In areas where nets are traditionally conical or are little used, people may not recognize pictures of rectangular nets. Another problem was drawing mosquitoes large enough to be seen and small enough to be recognizable as mosquitoes and not, for example, as birds. Further, some messages are difficult, if not impossible, to convey in pictures — for example, that people are happy to sleep under a net or that a net helps prevent malaria.

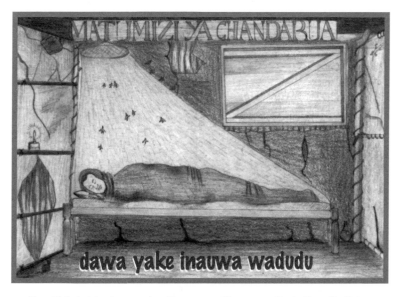

Figure 19. Bednet drawing as produced from a competition sponsored by the Rotary Net Project at the Ifakara Centre (Kilombero District, Tanzania). This illustration was drawn by 18-year-old Abrahami Majitanga.

It is also important to ensure exposure to print materials by distributing them widely. During the first net distribution in Bagamoyo, posters were displayed mainly at the distribution points, and booklets were given only to net buyers. When the effect of these materials was evaluated, it was decided that during subsequent rounds, posters should be displayed throughout villages and booklets should be distributed to all households.

Mass media

Little has been done to promote ITNs through the mass media. The Gambian national ITN program's experience with radio spots to promote net treatment is currently being evaluated. As shown by experience with the promotion of ORS, radio can be effective in promoting health.

Little social marketing has been done with ITNs in Africa: only one such program has been launched, in the Central African Republic (J. Berman, personal communication). Figure 20 shows a poster used by that project. Other countries also have a healthy advertising industry that should prove reliable for promoting ITNs once the distribution channels can be defined and the problem of re-treatment can be addressed.

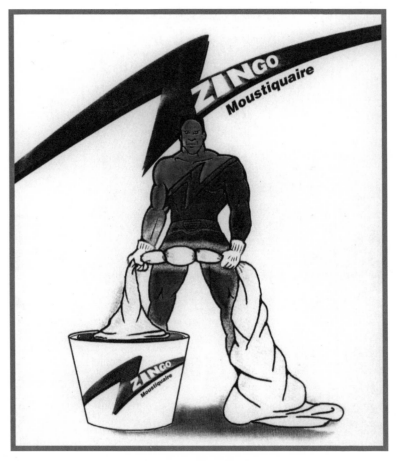

Figure 20. Poster from the ITN social-marketing program in the Central African Republic (Population Services International, PSI).

Conclusions

Most ITN projects have relied mainly on interpersonal contact for promotion, which largely reflects their small size and their level of funding. Much remains to be done to promote campaigns for larger programs.

The main lesson to be learned from ORS promotions is that the most effective approach is broad based, using a variety of media, to ensure that messages reach the target audience frequently and credibly. Theatre performances may not reach enough people frequently enough to be effective as a communication channel. Print materials must be developed carefully to suit the literacy level and iconographic range of the target community. Radio is likely to be important to national-level programs.

Recommendations

❖ Provide projects with information about all the essential elements presented in Table 15 to optimize implementation plans and optimize promotion of the intervention.

❖ Initially, for most sites, undertake fairly extensive formative research, as well as message testing and program evaluation: the amount of information available for most questions is limited, and it seems risky to generalize.

❖ Differentiate promotion activities and their evaluation into three conceptual areas: acquisition of nets or curtains, correct use by the target group, and re-treatment.

❖ For each conceptual area, define product, target audience, messages, and channels.

❖ Gather information in similar ways at individual sites so that it is more directly comparable. With experience, general patterns will appear.

❖ Identify the most cost-effective promotion and communication channels for each implementation model and location.

❖ Identify reinforcing (positive) and inhibiting (negative) messages for each location and audience.

❖ Establish the relative importance of a perceived reduction in nuisance biting and a perceived reduction in malaria as motivations for sustained ITN use. With experience, we can ascertain whether users will notice the reduction in malaria that results from ITN use and whether preventing disease will consequently become a stronger motivation for ITN use than reducing nuisance biting.

Chapter 5

Conclusions and Recommendations for Action

C. Lengeler, D. de Savigny, and J. Cattani

During the Dar es Salaam workshop, the definition and extent of operational research were discussed. It became clear that it is not always possible to separate recommendations for future research from more political recommendations to donor agencies and governments. Although this meeting was mainly concerned with research priorities (outlined in this chapter), it decided to list recommendations for political action as well.

Recommendations for Political Action

❖ Malaria prevention and control in African countries where the disease is endemic needs higher priority on the public-health agenda, consistent with the fact that it is the first cause of morbidity and mortality in these countries. Despite the practical problems interventions against malaria present, they have potential to improve child survival significantly.

❖ National governments, international agencies, and NGOs should cooperate to create a political environment that supports malaria control in general and preventive measures, such as ITNs, in particular. Pragmatic, flexible interaction among health-care providers should be encouraged.

❖ Concerted international action is required if strategic and technical guidelines on implementation of ITN programs are to be drawn up and disseminated, and these guidelines will require regular review. An international reference centre is needed to provide both information on the technical aspects of ITNs (insecticides, netting, dosage, resistance) and advice to governments on formulating relevant policies.

❖ Governments in areas with endemic malaria should create a favourable taxation environment based on analysis of the national market for either local net production or net imports.

❖ Institutions such as regional centres should be created for centralized procurement of netting and insecticide at the best possible price.

❖ Governments in areas with endemic malaria should issue guidelines on importing and using public-health-grade insecticides safely.

❖ Agencies implementing ITN programs should include operational research in their workplans and issue reports regularly. Ideally, the collaboration involved in research should make implementing agencies increasingly aware of the importance of applied operations research and should make researchers more responsive to specific program needs.

Recommendations for Future Research

The recommendations that follow consolidate and amplify those given in Chapters 2, 3, and 4. Some points overlap; others do not. This was done to distinguish the reviewers' opinions from those of the workshop participants.

Technology

The workshop participants reviewed the main technological research topics in detail and assigned highest priority to the following topics:

❖ Standardizing and improving tests for monitoring resistance to pyrethroids in mosquitoes; in the short term, improving procurement of susceptibility-testing and bioassay kits;

❖ Further work on determining optimal insecticide doses for the most popular types of netting (cotton, polyester, polyethylene, and nylon) and for various field situations;

❖ Developing simple tests for measuring pyrethroid doses on netting in routine program monitoring;

❖ Developing techniques for lengthening the re-treatment interval, such as incorporating long-acting insecticide into netting fibre;

❖ Developing new packaging for the most widely used insecticides, including a safe, inexpensive single-dose packet; and

❖ Refining dipping procedures to achieve a consistent target dose on netting with minimal wastage and environmental contamination; assessing the effectiveness and ease of application of other treatment procedures, such as spraying.

Overall, highest priority was given to development of new tests, either for assessing emerging resistance to pyrethroids in mosquitoes or for evaluating insecticide doses on netting. Materials (netting and insecticide) were also important. Stratification of participants (separating researchers from implementors and donors) revealed no major disagreement on priorities. Developing tools and techniques for monitoring mild and acute toxicity, entomological impact, or environmental impact did not receive high priority; measuring techniques for these parameters were deemed adequate.

Implementation

Participants recommended systematic study of various implementation models based on local conditions (actors, available structures and resources, political environment). Models could be defined as "pure" (exclusively private, governmental, or social marketing) or as "mixed" (two or more forms combined). Topics deemed worthy of investigation because of their potential for improvement of future ITN programs included the following:

❖ Pure and mixed implementation models with the prime objectives of feasibility, sustainability, and cost effectiveness — models include social marketing, private sector (commercial), PHC (government), nongovernmental, and intensified implementation in high-risk groups, such as young children and pregnant women;

❖ Integrating ITN activities with other health interventions, such as integrated management of the sick child and mother-and-child health;

❖ Developing specific decision-support models and other tools, such as political mapping, to support implementation models;

❖ Investigating new and established financing mechanisms designed for partial or total cost recovery within any of the proposed implementation models — this work should also cover traditional and innovative savings and credit systems and the effect of price on use of nets and insecticide; community-level financial management was seen as crucial and in need of more attention.

❖ Describing the effect of exemption from taxes and duties on net and insecticide availability and affordability; and

❖ Identify and describe key factors that influence program coverage and compliance.

Promotion

In the area of promotion, participants made the following recommendations:

❖ Stratify promotional activities and evaluation thereof into three conceptual areas: acquisition of nets or curtains, correct use by target group, and regular reimpregnation.

❖ Refine this stratification by defining, for each conceptual area, product, audience, communication channels, and the most relevant messages.

❖ Select the promotional approach that best suits the implementational approach; identify the most cost-effective communication channels for each model and each location.

❖ Identify reinforcing (positive) and inhibiting (negative) messages for each relevant setting and group.

❖ Examine what motivates households to acquire and use nets; the relationship between nuisance reduction and disease reduction; and how their relative importance changes over time.

❖ Establish optimal price structures for nets and insecticide and work toward resolving the conflict between affordability (which favours a low price) and perceived value and long-term sustainability (which favours a higher price).

Appendix 1

Acronyms and Abbreviations

CIF	carriage, insurance, and freight
DDP	delivered, duty paid
DDT	dichlorodiphenyltrichorethane
EC	emulsifiable concentrate
EHC	Environmental Health Criteria
EPI	Expanded Programme on Immunization
FOB	free on board
GNP	gross national product
IDRC	International Development Research Centre
ITN	insecticide-treated net
NGO	nongovernmental organization
NIBP	National Impregnated Bednet Programme
NIMR	Tanzanian National Institute of Medical Research
ORS	oral rehydration solution
PATH	Program for Appropriate Technology in Health
PHC	primary health care
s.l.	*sensu lato*
SP	synthetic pyrethroid
s.s.	*sensu stricto*
SSS	sugar–salt solution

TDR	UNDP/World Bank/WHO Special Programme for Research and Training in Tropical Diseases
UMCP	Urban Malaria Control Project (Dar es Salaam)
UNICEF	United Nations Children's Fund
WHO	World Health Organization
WP	wettable powder
WSS	water–sugar–salt (solution)

Appendix 2

Workshop Participants and Contributing Authors

Workshop Participants

Martin Alilio
National Institute for Medical
    Research
PO Box 9653
Dar es Salaam
Tanzania
Fax: (255 51) 30660

John Berman
Population Services International
1120 Nineteenth Street NW
Suite 600
Washington, DC 20036
USA
Fax: (202) 785 0120

Fred Binka
Navrongo Health Research Centre
Ministry of Health
PO Box 114
Navrongo
Ghana
Tel/fax: (233) 72 3425

Jacqueline Cattani
WHO/TDR
CH-1211 Geneva 27
Switzerland
Fax: (41 21) 791 4854

Lester Chitsulo
Ministry of Health
PO Box 30377
Capital City, Lilongwe
Malawi
Fax: (265) 783 109

Jean-Paul Clark
AID/AFR/ARTS/HHR
Agency for International
    Development
Bureau for Africa
Washington, DC 20523
USA
Fax: (703) 235 4466

Chris Curtis
London School of Hygiene and
    Tropical Medicine
Keppel Street
London WC1E 7HT
UK
Fax: (44 171) 636 8739

Don de Savigny
Health Sciences Division
IDRC
PO Box 8500
Ottawa, ON KIG 3H9
Canada
Fax: (613) 567 7748

Martinho Dgedge
Department of Blood Parasites
Instituto Nacional Saude
CP 264 Maputo
Mozambique
Fax: (258 1) 423726

Hokan Ekvall
Swedish Agency for Research
    Cooperation with Developing
    Countries
Box 16140
103 23 Stockholm
Sweden
Fax: (46 8) 622 5833

David Evans
WHO/TDR
CH-1211 Geneva 27
Switzerland
Fax: (41 21) 791 4854

Geraldine Farrell
Clonsilla Gorey Co.
Wexford
Ireland

Rachel Feilden
FBA
Riverside Cottage
Tellisford
Bath BA3 6RL
UK
Fax: (44 1373) 831 038

Timothy Freeman
2 Antrim Road
Avondale West
Harare
Zimbabwe
Fax: (263 4) 486 860

Christophe Codjo Gbaguidi
OSSD
BP 95 Savalou
Benin
Tel: (229) 54 0073

William Hawley
American Embassy/CDC
PO Box 30137
Nairobi
Kenya
Fax: (254 2) 714 608

Thomas van der Heijden
Netherlands Embassy
PO Box 9534
Dar es Salaam
United Republic of Tanzania
Fax: (255 51) 45189

Jenny Hill
Liverpool School of Tropical Medicine
Pembroke Pl
Liverpool L35QA
UK
Fax: (44 151) 707 1702

Wen Kilama
National Institute for Medical
    Research
PO Box 9653
Dar es Salaam
Tanzania
Fax: (255 51) 30660

Christian Lengeler
London School of Hygiene and
    Tropical Medicine
Keppel Street
London WC1E 7HT
UK
Fax: (44 171) 436 4230

Steve Lindsay
Danish Bilharziasis Laboratories
Jaegersborg Alle 1D
DK 2920 Charlottenlund
Denmark
Fax: (45 31) 62 61 21

Jo Lines
London School of Hygiene and
    Tropical Medicine
Keppel Street
London WC1E 7HT
UK
Fax: (44 171) 636 8739

Edith Lyimo
Ifakara Centre, NIMR
PO Box 53
Ifakara
Tanzania
Fax: (255 51) 30660

Stephen Magessa
National Institute for Medical
    Research
PO Box 9653
Dar es Salaam
Tanzania
Fax: (255 51) 30660

Abderhamane Sideye Maiga
Institut national de recherche en
    santé publique (INRSP)
Bamako
Mali
Fax: (223) 229 658

Sylvia Meek
Malaria Consortium
London School of Hygiene and
    Tropical Medicine
Keppel Street
London WC1E 7HT
UK
Fax: (44 171) 580 9075

Yvan Menard
PATH Canada
170 Laurier Avenue, W, Suite 902
Ottawa, ON K1P 5V5
Canada
Fax: (1 613) 230 8401

Omer Mensah
Centre Régional pour le
    développement et la santé
    (CREDESA)
BP 1822 Cotonou
Benin
Fax: (229) 30 12 88

Jane Miller
Mosquito Products Ltd
PO Box 72469
Dar es Salaam
Tanzania
Fax: (255 51) 75 670

Japhet Minjas
Department of Parasitology
    and Entomology
Muhimbili Medical Centre
PO Box 65001
Dar es Salaam
Tanzania
Fax: (255 51) 30 688

Dominic Mlula
Mosquito Products Ltd
PO Box 72469
Dar es Salaam
Tanzania
Fax: (255 51) 75 670

Fatma Mrisho
Ministry of Health
PO Box 9083
Dar es Salaam
Tanzania
Tel: (255 51) 236 76

Kopano Mukelabai
UNICEF Region Office
Kenya Country Office
PO Box 44145
Nairobi
Kenya
Fax: (254 2) 215 584

Halima Mwenesi
Kenya Medical Research Institute
Medical Research Centre
PO Box 20752
Nairobi
Kenya

Charles Oliver
USAID/G/HPN
Agency for International
   Development
Washington, DC 20523
USA
Fax: (703) 875 4686

Franco Pagnoni
Centre national de lutte contre
   le paludisme
01 BP 2208, Ouagadougou 01
Burkino Faso
Fax: (226) 31 04 77

Zul Premji
Department of Parasitology
   and Entomology
Muhimbili Medical Centre
PO Box 65001
Dar es Salaam
Tanzania
Fax: (255 51) 30 688

Selim Rashed
Centre for Tropical Diseases
Montreal General Hospital
1650 avenue des Cèdres, Room 787
Montréal, PQ H3G 1A4
Canada
Fax: (514) 933 9385

Catherine Reed
Malaria Unit
African Medical and Research
Foundation
PO Box 30125
Nairobi
Kenya
Fax: (254 2) 506 112

Clive Shiff
Johns Hopkins University
615 N Wolfe Street
Baltimore, MD 21205
USA
Fax: (410) 614 1419

Eliab Some
Malaria Unit
African Medical and Research
Foundation
PO Box 30125
Nairobi
Kenya
Fax: (254 2) 506 112

Timothy Stone
PATH Canada
170 Laurier Avenue W, Suite 902
Ottawa, ON K1P 5V5
Canada
Fax: (613) 230 8401

Yves Traoré
Centre Muraz
01 BP 153, Bobo-Dioulasso
Burkina Faso
Fax: (226) 970 099

Peter Winch
Johns Hopkins University
615 N Wolfe Street
Baltimore, MD 21205
USA
Fax: (410) 614 1419

Susan Zimicki
21 South Strawberry St 6D
Philadelphia, PA 19106
USA
Tel/fax: (1 215) 922 2584

Contributing Authors

Jacqueline Cattani
UNDP/World Bank/WHO Special
    Programme for Research and
    Training in Tropical Diseases
World Health Organization
1211 Geneva 27
Switzerland
e-mail: cattani@who.ch
Tel: (41 22) 791 3737
Fax: (41 22) 791 4854

Don de Savigny
International Development
    Research Centre
PO Box 8500
Ottawa, ON K1G 3H9
Canada
e-mail: ddesavigny@idrc.ca
Tel: (613) 236 6163
Fax: (613) 567 7748

Rachel Feilden
FBA Health Systems Analysts
Riverside Cottage
Tellisford
Bath BA3 6RL
UK
Tel: (44 1373) 830 322
Fax: (44 1373) 831 038

Christian Lengeler
Swiss Tropical Institute
PO Box
CH-4002 Basel
Switzerland
e-mail: lengeler@ubaclu.unibas.ch
Tel: (41 61) 284 8221
Fax: (41 61) 271 7951

Jo Lines
Vector Biology and Epidemiology
    Unit
London School of Hygiene and
    Tropical Medicine
Keppel Street
London WC1E 7HT
UK
e-mail: jlines@lshtm.ac.uk
Tel: (44 171) 927 2461
Fax: (44 171) 636 8739

Susan Zimicki
Annenberg School of
    Communications
University of Pennsylvania
Philadelphia, PA
USA
e-mail: szimicki@ad.com
Tel/fax: (215) 898 2024

Bibliography

Agyepong, I.A. 1992. Malaria: Ethnomedical perceptions and practice in an Adangbe farming community and implications for control. Social Science and Medicine, 35(2), 131–137.

Aikins, M.K. 1995. Cost-effectiveness analysis of insecticide-impregnated mosquito nets (bednets) used as a malaria control measure: a study from The Gambia. University of London, London, UK. PhD thesis. 324 pp.

Aikins, M.K.; Pickering, H.A.; Alonso, P.L.; d'Alessandro, U.; Linsay, S.W.; Todd, J.; Greenwood, B.M. 1993. A malaria control trial using insecticide-treated bednets and targeted chemoprophylaxis in a rural area of The Gambia, West Africa. 4. Perceptions of the causes of malaria and of its treatment and prevention in the study area. Transactions of the Royal Society of Tropical Medicine and Hygiene, 87(suppl. 2), 25–30.

Aikins, M.K.; Pickering, H.; Greenwood, B.M. 1994. Attitudes to malaria, traditional practices and bednets (mosquito nets) as vector control measures: a comparative study in five West African countries. Journal of Tropical Medicine and Hygiene, 97, 81–86.

Alonso, P.L.; Lindsay, S.W.; Armstrong, J.R.M.; Konteh, M.; Hill, A.G.; David, P.H.; Fegan, G.; DeFrancisco, A.; Hall, A.J.; Shenton, F.C.; Cham, K.; Greenwood, B.M. 1991. The effect of insecticide treated bed nets on mortality of Gambian children. Lancet, 337, 1499–1502.

Alonso, P.L.; Lindsay, S.W.; Armstrong-Schellenberg, J.R.M.; Keita, K.; Gomez, P.; Shenton, F.C.; Hill, A.G.; David, P.H.; Fegan, G.; Cham, K.; Greenwood, B.M. 1993. A malaria control trial using insecticide-treated bednets and targeted chemoprophylaxis in a rural area of The Gambia, West Africa. 6. The impact of the interventions on mortality and morbidity from malaria. Transactions of the Royal Society of Tropical Medicine and Hygiene, 87(suppl. 2), 37–44.

Alonso, P.L.; Lindsay, S.W.; Armstrong-Schellenberg, J.R.M.; Konteh, M.; Keita, K.; Marshall, C.; Phillips, A.; Cham, K.; Greenwood, B.M. 1993. A malaria control trial using insecticide-treated bednets and targeted chemoprophylaxis in a rural area of The Gambia, West Africa. 5. Design and implementation of the trial. Transactions of the Royal Society of Tropical Medicine and Hygiene, 87(suppl. 2), 31–36.

Ardener, S. 1978. The comparative study of rotating savings and credit associations. Journal of the Royal Anthropological Society Institute, 94, 201–228.

Ardener, S.; Burman, S., ed. 1995. Money-go-rounds: The importance of ROSCAs for women. Berg Publishers, Oxford, UK. 320 pp.

Bagamoyo Bed Net Project. 1992. Annual report. Muhimbili Medical Centre, Dar es Salaam, Tanzania. 44 pp.

Beach, R.F.; Ruebush, T.K, II; Sexton, J.D.; Bright, P.L.; Hightower, A.W.; Breman, J.G.; Mount, D.L.; Oloo, A.J. 1993. Effectiveness of permethrin impregnated bednets and curtains for malaria control in a holoendemic area of western Kenya. American Journal of Tropical Medicine and Hygiene, 49, 290–300.

Bennett, S.; Ngalande-Banda, E. 1994. Public and private roles in health: a review and analysis of experience in sub-Saharan Africa. World Health Organization, Geneva, Switzerland. WHO/SHS/CC/94.1. 42 pp.

Binka, F.N.; Kubaje, A.; Adjuik, M.; Williams, L.; Lengeler, C.; Maude, G.H.; Armah, G.E.; Kajihara, B.; Adiamah, J.H.; Smith, P.G. 1996. Impact of permethrin impregnated bednets on child mortality in Kassena–Nankana District, Ghana: a randomized controlled trial. Tropical Medicine and International Health, 1(2), 147–154.

Bomann, W. 1996. How safe are pyrethroid-treated mosquito nets? An evaluation based on the example of Solfac EW 050. Public Health (Bayer), 12, 30–35.

Bouman, F.J.A. 1978. Indigenous savings and credit societies in the Third World: a message. Savings and Development, 4.1, 181–219.

Bradley, A.K.; Greenwood, B.M.; Greenwood, A.M.; Marsh, K.; Byass, P.; Tullock, S; Hayes, R. 1986. Bednets (mosquito nets) and morbidity from malaria. Lancet, 336(2), 204–207.

Bradley, D.J. 1991. Morbidity and mortality at Pare-Taweta, Kenya and Tanzania, 1954–66: the effects of a period of malaria control. In Feachem, R.G.; Jamison, D., ed., Disease and mortality in sub-Saharan Africa. Oxford University Press, Oxford, UK. pp. 248–262.

Brieger, W. 1990. Mass media and health communication in rural Nigeria. Health Policy and Planning, 5(1), 77–81.

Campbell, J.G.; Shrestha, R.; Stone, L. 1979. The use and misuse of social science research in Nepal. Research Centre for Nepal and Asian Studies, Tribhuvan University, Kirtipur, Kathmandu, Nepal. 88 pp.

Carme, B.; Koulengana, P.; Nzambi, A.; Guillodubodan, H. 1992. Current practices for the prevention and treatment of malaria in children and in pregnant women in the Brazzaville region (Congo). Annals of Tropical Medicine and Parasitology, 86(4), 319–322.

Carnevale, P.; Coosemans, M. 1995. Some operational aspects of the use of personal protection methods against malaria at individual and community levels. Annales de la Société Belge de médecine tropicale, 75, 81–103.

Carnevale, P.; Robert, V.; Boudin, C.; Halna, J.-M.; Pasart, L.; Gazin, P.; Richard, A.; Mouchet, J. 1988. La lutte contre le paludisme par des moustiquaires imprégnées de pyréthroides au Burkina Faso. Bulletin de la Société de pathologie exotique, 81, 832–846.

Carnevale, P.; Robert, V.; Snow, R.W.; Curtis, C.; Richard, A.; Boudin, C.; Pazart, L.-H.; Halna, J.M.; Mouchet, J. 1991. L'impact des moustiquaires imprégnées sur la prévalence et la morbidité lié au paludisme en Afrique subsaharienne. Annales de la Société Belge de médecine tropicale, 71 (suppl. 1), 127–150.

Carr, D.; Way, A. 1994. Women's lives and experiences: a decade of research findings from the Demographic and Health Surveys Programme. Macro International, Calverton, MD, USA. 92 pp.

Charlwood, J.D. 1986. A differential response to mosquito nets by *Anopheles* and *Culex* mosquitoes from Papua New Guinea. Transactions of the Royal Society of Tropical Medicine and Hygiene, 80, 958–960.

Charlwood, J.D.; Dagoro, H. 1989. Collateral effects of bednets impregnated with permethrin against bedbugs (Cimicidae) in Papua New Guinea. Transactions of the Royal Society of Tropical Medicine and Hygiene, 83, 261.

Charlwood, J.D.; Graves, P.M. 1987. The effect of permethrin-impregnated bednets on a population of *Anopheles farauti* in coastal Papua New Guinea. Medical and Veterinary Entomology, 1, 319–327.

Cheng H.; Yang W.; Kang W.; Liu C. 1995. Large-scale spraying of bednets to control mosquito vectors and malaria in Sichuan, China. Bulletin of the World Health Organization, 73(3), 321–328.

Chitsulo, L.; Ettling, M.; Macheso, A.; Steketee, R.; Schultz, L.; Ziwa, C. 1992. Malaria in Malawi: knowledge, attitudes and practices. USAID Contract No. DPE-DPE-5948-Q-9030-00 to Medical Service Corporation International, Arlington, VA, USA. 45 pp. Vector Biology Control Report No. 82240.

Choi, H.W.; Breman, J.G.; Teutsch S.M.; Liu, S.; Hightower, A.W.; Sexton, J.D. 1995. The effectiveness of insecticide-impregnated bed nets in reducing cases of malaria infection: a meta-analysis of published results. American Journal of Tropical Medicine and Hygiene, 52(5), 377–382.

Chowdhury, A.M.R.; Vaughan, J.P.; Adel, F.H. 1988. Use and safety of homemade rehydration solutions: an epidemiological evaluation from Bangladesh. International Journal of Epidemiology, 17, 655–665.

Ciszewscki, R.L.; Harvey, P.D. 1994. The effect of price increases on contraceptive sales in Bangladesh. Journal of Biosocial Science, 26(1), 25–35.

Curtis, C.F. 1987. Genetic aspects of selection for resistance. *In* Ford, M.G.; Holloman, D.W.; Khambay, B.P.S.; Sawicki, S.M. ed., Combating resistance to xenobiotics. Ellis Horwood, Chichester, UK. pp. 150–161.

Curtis, C.F. 1992a. Personal protection methods against vectors of disease. Review of Medical and Veterinary Entomology, 80, 543–553.

———— 1992b. Spraying bednets with deltamethrin in Sichuan, China: abstracts of selected Chinese papers and discussion (with new data). Tropical Diseases Bulletin, 89, R1–R6.

———— 1992c. Impregnated mosquito nets. Footsteps, 10, 14–15.

———— 1992d. Workshop on bednets at the International Congress of Tropical Medicine. Japanese Journal of Sanitary Zoology, 44, 65–68.

Curtis, C.F.; Hill, N.; Kasim, K. 1993. Are there effective resistance management strategies for vectors of human disease? Biological Journal of the Linnean Society, 48, 3–18.

Curtis, C.F.; Lines, J.D.; Carnevale, P.; Robert, V.; Boudin, C.; Halna, J.-M.; Pazart, L.; Gazin, P.; Richard, A.; Mouchet, J.; Charlwood, J.D.; Graves, P.M.; Hossain, M.I.; Kurihara, T.; Ichimori, K.; Li Zuzi; Lu Baolin; Majori, G.; Sabatinelli, G.; Coluzzi, M.; Njunwa, K.J.; Wilkes, T.J.; Snow, R.W.; Lindsay, S.W. 1991. Impregnated bed nets and curtains against malaria mosquitoes. *In* Curtis, C.F., ed., Control of disease vectors in the community. Wolfe Publishing, London, UK. pp. 5–46.

Curtis, C.F.; Myamba, J.; Wilkes, T.J. 1992. Various pyrethroids on bednets and curtains. Memorias del Instituto Oswaldo Cruz, 87(suppl. 3), 363–370.

———1996. Comparison of different insecticides and fabrics for anti-mosquito bednets and curtains. Medical and Veterinary Entomology, 10, 1–11.

Curtis, C.F.; Wilkes, T.J.; Myamba, J.; Chambika, C. 1994. Insecticide impregnated bednets: Comparison of different insecticides and fabrics (abstract). Transactions of the Royal Society of Tropical Medicine and Hygiene, 88, 373.

d'Alessandro, U.; Aikins, M.K.; Langerock, P.; Bennet, S.; Greenwood, B.M. 1994. Nationwide survey of bednet use in rural Gambia. Bulletin of the World Health Organization, 72(3), 391–394.

d'Alessandro, U.; Olaleye, B.O.; McGuire, W.; Langerock, P.; Bennett, S.; Aikins, M.K.; Thomson, M.C.; Cham, M.K.; Cham, B.A.; Greenwood, B.M. 1995. Mortality and morbidity from malaria in Gambian children after the introduction of an impregnated bed net programme. Lancet, 345, 479–483.

Desfontaine, M.; Gelas, H.; Cabon, J.; Goghomou, A.; Kouka Bemba, D.; Carnevale, P. 1990. Évaluation des pratiques et des coûts de lutte antivectorielle à l'échelon familial en Afrique centrale. II. Ville de Douala (Cameroun), juillet 1988. Annales de la Société belge de médecine tropicale, 70, 137–144.

Desfontaine, M.; Gelas, H.; Goghomu, A.; Kouka-Bemba, D; Carnevale, P. 1989. Évaluation des pratiques et des coûts de lutte antivectorielle à l'échelon familial en Afrique centrale. I. Ville de Yaoundé (mars 1988). Bulletin de la Société de pathologie exotique, 82, 558–565.

Dollimore, L. 1993. Safe packaging and labelling of pesticides. *In* Forget, G.; Goodman, T.; de Villiers, A., ed., Impact of pesticide use on health in developing countries: Proceedings of a symposium held in Ottawa, ON, Canada, 17–20 September 1990. International Development Research Centre, Ottawa, ON, Canada. pp. 121–132.

Elder, J.; Geller, S.; Touchette, P.; Foote, D.; Smith, W. 1987. The Healthcom Project and the behavioral management of diarrhoea. International Quarterly of Community Health Education, 8(3), 201–211.

Elissa, N.; Curtis, C.F. 1995. Evaluation of different formulations of deltamethrin in comparison with permethrin for impregnation of netting. Pesticide Science, 44, 363–367.

Ettling, M.; McFarland, D.A.; Schultz, L.J.; Chitsulo, L. 1994. Economic impact of malaria in low-income households. Tropical Medicine and Parasitology, 45, 74–79.

Evans, P. 1994. Community knowledge, attitudes and practices: urban mosquitoes and their sustainable control. University of Exeter, Exeter, UK. PhD thesis. 289 pp.

Feilden, R. 1991. Use of cost-effectiveness analysis in three countries in Eastern and Southern Africa region: report of a consultancy for UNICEF Eastern and Southern Africa Regional Office. UNICEF, Nairobi, Kenya. 24 pp.

Foote, D. 1985. The mass media and health practices evaluation in The Gambia: a report of the major findings. Applied Communications Technologies, Menlo Park, CA, USA. 111 pp.

Geertz, C. 1962. The rotating credit associations: a "middle rung" in development. Economic Development and Cultural Change, 1.3, 241–263.

Gilles, H.M. 1993. Epidemiology of malaria. In Gilles, H.M.; Warrell, D.A., ed., Bruce Chwatt's essential malariology. E. Arnold, London, UK. pp. 124–163.

Gillett, J.D. 1985. The behaviour of Homo sapiens, the forgotten factor in the transmission of tropical disease. Transactions of the Royal Society of Tropical Medicine and Hygiene, 79, 12–20.

GOK–UNICEF (Ministry of Health, Kenya – United Nations Children's Fund). 1990. Malaria Control/Bamako Initiative Programme, East Koguta Location, Upper Nyakach Division, Kisumu District. CHWs training on malaria control at Sigoti from 16.10.90 to 29.10.90. UNICEF, Nairobi, Kenya. 21 pp.

———— 1992. Financial management within Bamako Initiative projects: a training manual for district and divisional health management teams. UNICEF Nairobi, Kenya. 22 pp.

Graeff, J.A.; Elder, J.P.; Booth, E.M., ed. 1993. Communication for health and behavior change. Jossey-Bass Publishers, San Francisco, CA, USA. 213 pp.

Green, L.W.; Kreuter, M.W.; Deeds, S.G.; Partridge, K.B.; Bartlett, E., ed. 1980. Health education planning — a diagnostic approach. Mayfield Publishing, Palo Alto, CA, USA. 153 pp.

Greenwood, B.M. 1994. The Gambian national impregnated bednet programme. Progress report to WHO/TDR. World Health Organization, Geneva, Switzerland. 44 pp.

Guiguemde, T.R.; Dao, F.; Curtis, V.; Traore, A.; Sondo, B.; Testa, J.; Ouedraogo, J.B. 1994. Household expenditure on malaria prevention and treatment for families in the town of Bobo-Dioulasso, Burkina Faso. Transactions of the Royal Society of Tropical Medicine and Hygiene, 88, 285–287.

Gyapong, M.; Gyapong, J.O.; Amankwa, J.A.; Asedem, J.T.; Sory, E.K. 1992. "We have been looking for something like this for a long time": acceptability of the use of insecticide impregnated bednets in an area of low bednet usage. Health Research Unit, Ministry of Health, Accra, Ghana. 18 pp.

Haaland, A. 1984. Pretesting communication material — a manual for trainers and supervisors. UNICEF, Rangoon, Myanmar. 62 pp.

Harper, P.A.; Lisansky, E.T.; Sasse, B.E. 1947. Malaria and other insect-borne diseases in the South Pacific campaign 1942–45. American Journal of Tropical Medicine and Hygiene 27(suppl.), 1.

Harvey, P.D. 1994. The impact of condom prices on sales in social marketing programs. Studies in Family Planning, 25(1), 52–58.

He F.; Wang S.; Liu L.; Chen S.; Zhang Z.; Sun J. 1989. Clinical manifestations and diagnosis of acute pyrethroid poisoning. Archives of Toxociology, 63, 54–58.

Hii, J.L.; Kanai, L.; Foligela, A.; Kan, S.K.; Burkot, T.R.; Wirtz, R.A. 1993. Impact of permethrin-impregnated mosquito nets compared with DDT housespraying against malaria transmission by An. farauti and An. punctulatus in the Solomon Islands. Medical and Veterinary Entomology, 7, 333–338.

Hill, J. 1990. KAP survey related to malaria illness and the mosquito vector in the pilot Malaria Control Programme area of west Kabar. UNICEF, Nairobi, Kenya. 22 pp.

———— 1991. Evaluation of impregnated bednets distributed as part of the GOK/UNICEF malaria control programme in west Kabar. UNICEF, Nairobi, Kenya. 43 pp.

———— 1992. Manual for the DHMT and field workers in community-based malaria control. UNICEF, Nairobi, Kenya. 37 pp.

Ho C.; Chou T.; Chen T.; Hsueh A. 1962. The Anopheles hyrcanus group and its relation to malaria in east China. China Medical Journal, 81, 71–78

Hornik, R. 1988. Development communication. Longman, New York, NY, USA. pp. 118–137.

Hornik, R.; Sankar, P.; Huntington, D.; Matsebula, G.; Mndzebele, A.; Magongo, B. 1986. Communication for diarrheal disease control: evaluation of the Swaziland program 1984–85. Academy for Educational Development, Washington, DC, USA. 112 pp.

Hossain, M.I.; Curtis, C.F. 1989. Permethrin-impregnated bednets: behavioural and killing affects against mosquitoes. Medical and Veterinary Entomology, 3, 367–376.

Hossain, M.I.; Curtis, C.F.; Heekin, J.P. 1989. Assays of permethrin-impregnated fabrics and bioassays with mosquitoes. Bulletin of Entomological Research, 79, 299–308.

Ismail, I.A.H.; Pinichpongse, S.; Boonrasri, P. 1978. Responses of An. minimus to DDT spraying in a cleared forested foothill area in central Thailand. Acta Tropica, 69, 69–82.

Jaenson, T.G.T.; Gomes, M.J.; Barreto dos Santos, R.C.; Petrarca, V.; Fortini, D.; Evora, J.; Crato, J. 1994. Control of endophagic *Anopheles* mosquitoes and human malaria in Guinea Bissau, West Africa by use of permethrin-treated bed nets. Transactions of the Royal Society of Tropical Medicine and Hygiene, 88, 620–624.

Jana-Kara, B.R.; Adak, T.; Curtis, C.F.; Sharma, V.P. 1994. Laboratory studies of different pyrethroid-netting combinations to kill mosquitoes. Indian Journal of Malariology, 31, 1–11.

Jana-Kara, B.R.; Jihullah, W.A.; Shahi, B.; Dev, V.; Curtis, C.F.; Sharma, V.P. 1995. Deltamethrin impregnated bednets against *Anopheles minimus* transmitted malaria in Assam, India. Journal of Tropical Medicine and Hygiene, 98, 73–83.

Karch, S.; Garin, B.; Asidi, N.; Manzambi, Z.; Salaun, J.J.; Mouchet, J. 1993. Moustiquaires impregnées contre le paludisme au Zaire. Annales de la Société belge de médecine tropicale, 73, 37–53.

Kenya, P.R.; Gatiti, S.; Muthami, L.N.; Agwanda, R.; Mwenesi, H.A.; Katsivo, M.N.; Omondi-Odhiambo; Surrow, A.; Juma, R.; Ellison, R.H.; Cooper, G.; van Andel, F. 1990. Oral rehydration therapy and social marketing in rural Kenya. Social Science and Medicine, 31(9), 979–987.

Kere, N.K.; Parkinson, A.D.; Samrawickrema, W.A. 1993. The effect of permethrin impregnated bednets on the incidence of *Plasmodium falciparum* in children of north Guadalcanal, Solomon Islands. Southeast Asian Journal of Tropical Medicine and Public Health, 24, 130–137.

Kroeger, A. 1985. Response errors and other problems of health interview surveys in developing countries. World Health Statistics Quarterly, 38, 15–21.

Kroeger, A.; Alarçon, J., ed. 1993. Malaria en Ecuador y Perú y estrategias alternativas de control. Ediciónes Abya-Yala, Quito, Ecuador. 316 pp.

Kroeger, A.; Mancheno, M.; Alarçon, J.; Pesse, K. 1995. Insecticide impregnated mosquito nets for malaria control: varying experiences from Ecuador and Peru, concerning their acceptability and effectiveness. American Journal of Tropical Medicine and Hygiene, 53(4), 313–323.

Kroeger, A.; Mancheno, M.; Ruiz, W.; Estrella, E., ed. 1991. Malaria y *Leishmaniasis cutanea* en Ecuador. Museo Nacional de Medicina, Quito, Ecuador; University of Heidelberg, Germany; Ediciónes Abya-Yala, Quito, Ecuador. 374 pp.

Kuate Defo, B. 1995. Epidemiology and control of infant and early childhood malaria: a competing risk analysis. International Journal of Epidemiology, 24(1), 204–217.

Ladonni, H.; Bomet, R.O.; Crampton, J.; Townson, H. 1990. Genetics of pyrethroid resistance in the mosquito *An. stephensi*. Transactions of the Royal Society of Tropical Medicine and Hygiene, 84, 459.

Last, J.M. 1995. A dictionary of epidemiology. Oxford University Press, Oxford, UK. 180 pp.

Lengeler, C.; Lines, J.D.; Cattani, J.A.; Feilden, R.; Zimicki, S.; de Savigny, D. 1996. Promoting operational research on insecticide-treated netting: a joint TDR/IDRC initiative and call for research proposals. Tropical Medicine and International Health, 1(2), 273–276.

Lengeler, C.; Snow, R.W. 1996. From efficacy to effectiveness: the case of insecticide-treated bed nets in Africa. Bulletin of the World Health Organization, 74 (3).

Li Z.; Zhang M.; Wu Y.; Zhong B.; Lin G.; Huang H. 1989. Trial of deltamethrin impregnated bednets for the control of malaria transmitted by An. sinensis and An. anthropophagus. American Journal of Tropical Medicine and Hygiene, 40, 356–359.

Liambila, W.; Maneno, J.; Hill, J. 1994. A practical guide to the planning and implementation of the Bamako Initiative in Kenya. UNICEF, Nairobi, Kenya. 33 pp.

Lindsay, S.W.; Gibson, M.E. 1988. Bednets revisited — old idea, new angle. Parasitology Today, 4(10), 270–272.

Lindsay, S.W.; Adiamah, J.H.; Armstrong, J.R.M. 1992. The effect of permethrin-impregnated bednets on house entry by mosquitoes in The Gambia. Bulletin of Entomological Research, 82, 49–55.

Lindsay, S.W.; Adiamah, J.H.; Miller, J.E.; Armstrong J.R.M. 1991. Pyrethroid-treated bednets' effects on mosquitoes of the Anopheles gambiae complex in The Gambia. Medical and Veterinary Entomology, 5, 477–483.

Lindsay, S.W.; Alonso, P.L.; Armstrong-Schellenberg, J.R.M.; Hemingway, J.; Adiamah, J.H.; Shenton, F.C.; Jawara, M.; Greenwood, B.M. 1993. A malaria control trial using insecticide-treated bednets and targeted chemoprophylaxis in a rural area of The Gambia, West Africa. 7. Impact of permethrin-impregnated bednets on malaria vectors. Transactions of the Royal Society of Tropical Medicine and Hygiene, 87(suppl. 2), 45–51.

Lindsay, S.W.; Hossain, M.I.; Bennett, S.; Curtis, C.F. 1991. Preliminary studies on the insecticidal activity and wash-fastness of twelve pyrethroid treatments impregnated into bednetting assayed against mosquitoes. Pesticide Sciences, 32, 397–411.

Lindsay, S.W.; Snow, R.W.; Armstrong, J.R.M.; Greenwood, B.M. 1989. Permethrin-impregnated bednets reduce nuisance arthropods in Gambia houses. Medical and Veterinary Entomology, 3, 377–383.

Lindsay, S.W.; Snow, R.W.; Broomfield, G.L.; Semega Janneh, M.; Wirtz, R.A.; Greenwood, B.M. 1989. Impact of permethrin-treated bednets on malaria transmission by the Anopheles gambiae complex in The Gambia. Medical and Veterinary Entomology, 3, 263–271.

Lines, J.D. 1988. Do agricultural insecticides select for insecticide resistance in mosquitoes? A look at the evidence. Parasitology Today, 4(suppl.), S17–S20.

Lines, J.D.; Myamba, J.; Curtis, C.F. 1987. Experimental hut trials of permethrin impregnated mosquito nets and eave curtains against malaria vectors in Tanzania. Medical and Veterinary Entomology, 1, 37–51.

Louis, J.P.; Desfontaine, M.; Trebucq, A.; Gelas, H.; Carnevale, P. 1990. Lutte antivectorielle et prise en charge du paludisme-maladie à l'échelon familial: évolution méthodologique de l'évaluation des pratiques et des coûts. OCEAC, Yaoundé, Cameroon. 8 pp.

Louis, J.P.; Le Goff, G.; Trebucq, A.; Migliani, R.; Louis, F.J.; Robert, V.; Carnevale, P. 1992. Faisabilité de la stratégie de lutte par moustiquaires de lit imprégnées d'insecticide rémanent en zone rurale au Cameroun. Annales de la Société belge de médecine tropicale, 72, 189–195.

Luo D.-P.; La D.; Yao R.; Li P.; Huo X.; Li A.; Wen L.; Ge C.; Zhang S.; Huo H.; Shang L. 1994. Alphamethrin-impregnated bed nets for malaria and mosquito control in China. Transactions of the Royal Society of Tropical Medicine and Hygiene, 88, 625–628.

Lyimo, E.O.; Msuya, F.H.M.; Rwegoshora, R.T.; Nicholson, E.A.; Mnzava, A.E.P.; Lines, J.D.; Curtis, C.F. 1991. Trial of pyrethroid impregnated bednets in an area of Tanzania holoendemic for malaria. Part 3. Effects on the prevalence of malaria parasitaemia and fever. Acta Tropica, 49, 157–163.

MacCormack, C.P.; Snow, R.W. 1986. Gambian cultural preferences in the use of insecticide-impregnated bed nets. Journal of Tropical Medicine and Hygiene, 89, 295–302.

MacCormack, C.P.; Snow, R.W.; Greenwood, B.M. 1989. Use of insecticide-impregnated bed nets in Gambian primary health care: economic aspects. Bulletin of the World Health Organization, 67(2), 209–214.

Magesa, S.M.; Aina, O.; Curtis, C.F. 1994. Detection of pyrethroid resistance in Anopheles mosquitoes. Bulletin of the World Health Organization, 72, 737–740.

Magesa, S.M.; Wilkes, T.J.; Mnzava, A.E.P.; Njunwa, K.J.; Myamba, J.; Kivuyo, M.V.P.; Hill, N.; Lines, J.D.; Curtis, C.F. 1991. Trial of pyrethroid impregnated bednets in an area of Tanzania holoendemic for malaria. Part 2. Effects on the malaria vector population. Acta Tropica, 49, 97–108.

Makemba, A.M.; Winch, P.J.; Kamazima, S.R.; Makame, V.; Sengo, F.; Lubega, P.B.; Minjas, J.N.; Shiff, C.J. 1995. Implementation of a community-based system for the sale, distribution and insecticide impregnation of mosquito nets in Bagamoyo District, Tanzania. Health Policy and Planning, 10(1), 50–59.

Malcolm, C.A. 1988. Current status of pyrethroid resistance in anophelines. Parasitology Today, 4(suppl.), S13–S15.

Management Sciences for Health. 1981. Managing drug supply. Management Sciences for Health, Boston, MA, USA. 585 pp.

Marbiah, N.T. 1995. Control of disease due to perennially transmitted malaria in children in a rural area of Sierra Leone. University of London, London, UK. PhD thesis. 315 pp.

Marchand, R.P. 1994. Towards sustainable malaria control in Vietnam: background, organisation and progress results of district-scale trials with impregnated bednets. Medical Committee Netherlands–Viet Nam, Amsterdam, the Netherlands. 48 pp.

Marsh, V. 1994. A report on a ITB teaching programme in primary schools. KEMRI Kilifi Unit, Kilifi, Kenya. 20 pp.

McBean, G. 1989. Rethinking visual literacy — helping pre-literates learn. UNICEF, Kathmandu, Nepal. 25 pp.

McDivitt, J.; Myers, C. 1987. Preliminary results from the follow-up survey in The Gambia. Applied Communication Technology, Menlo Park, CA, USA. 27 pp.

Meek, S.R.; Kamwi, R. 1991. A survey of the knowledge, attitudes and practice of the population of Ovamboland, northwest Namibia related to malaria and of the effectiveness of the residual spraying programme. WHO, Windhoek, Namibia. 13 pp.

Miller, J.E. 1990. Laboratory and field studies of insecticide impregnated fibres from mosquito control. University of London, London, UK. PhD thesis. 287 pp.

———— 1994a. Relative efficacy of three pyrethroid insecticides for treating mosquito bednets. Pesticide Outlook, 5, 23–25.

———— 1994b. Can pyriproxyfen (an insect growth regulator) be used to prevent selection of permethrin resistance by impregnated bednets? Transactions of the Royal Society of Tropical Medicine and Hygiene, 88, 281.

Miller, J.E.; Lindsay, S.W.; Armstrong, J.R.M. 1991. Experimental hut trials of bednets impregnated with synthetic pyrethroid or organophosphate insecticide for mosquito control in The Gambia. Medical and Veterinary Entomology, 5, 465–476.

Miller, J.E.; Lindsay, S.W.; Armstrong-Schellenberg, J.R.M.; Adiamah, J.; Jawara, M.; Curtis, C.F. 1995. Village trial of bednets impregnated with wash-resistant permethrin compared with other pyrethroid formulations. Medical and Veterinary Entomology, 9, 43–49.

Mills, A.; Fox-Rushby, J.; Aikins, M.; d'Alessandro, U.; Cham, K.; Greenwood, B. 1994. Financing mechanisms for village activities in The Gambia and their implications for financing insecticide for bednet impregnation. Journal of Tropical Medicine and Hygiene, 97, 325–332.

Miracle, M.P.; Miracle, D.S.; Cohen, L. 1980. Informal savings mobilisation in Africa. Economic Development and Cultural Change, 1980, 701–724.

Molineaux, L.; Gramiccia, G., ed. 1980. The Garki project. World Health Organization, Geneva, Switzerland. 311 pp.

Muller, O.; Quinones, M.; Cham, K.; Aikins, M.; Greenwood, B. 1994. Detecting permethrin on nets. Lancet, 344, 1699–1700.

Munasinghe, C.S. 1994. An evaluation of the comparative efficacy of permethrin, lambdacyhalothrin, and bendiocarb impregnated house curtains against *Culex quinquefasciatus* in Matra, Sri Lanka. University of London, London, UK. MSc thesis. 47 pp.

Mutinga, M.J.; Mnzava, A.; Kiokoti, R.; Nyamori, M.; Ngindu, A.M. 1993. Malaria prevalence and morbidity in relation to the use of permethrin-treated wall cloths in Kenya. East African Medical Journal, 70, 756–762.

Mutinga, M.J.; Mutero, C.M.; Basimike, M.; Ngindu, A.M. 1992. The use of permethrin-impregnated wall-cloth (Mbu-cloth) for control of vectors of malaria and leishmaniases in Kenya. 1. Effect on mosquito populations. Insect Science and Its Applications, 13, 151–158.

Mwenesi, H.A.; Harpham, T.; Marsh, K.; Snow, R.W. 1995. Perceptions of symptoms of severe childhood malaria among Mijikenda and Luo residents of coastal Kenya. Journal of Biosocial Science, 27, 235–244.

Nagle, L.C.S. 1994. Experimental hut studies on the ability of bednets impregnated with permethrin to kill mosquitoes in The Gambia. University of London, London, UK. MSc thesis, 82 pp.

Nevill, C.G.; Some, E.S.; Mung'ala, V.O.; Mutemi, W.; New, L.; Marsh, K.; Lengeler, C.; Snow, R.W. 1996. Insecticide treated bednets reduce mortality and severe morbidity from malaria among children on the Kenyan coast. Tropical Medicine and International Health, 1(2), 139–146.

NIBP (National Impregnated Bednet Programme). 1993a. Report on the 1992 bednet impregnation process. NIBP, MRC Fajara, The Gambia. 18 pp.

——————— 1993b. Report on the implementation component of the National Impregnated Bednet Programme. NIBP, MRC Fajara, The Gambia. 21 pp.

NIH–NCI (National Institute of Health — National Cancer Institute). 1989. Making health communication programs work. A planners guide. NIH–NCI, Baltimore, MD, USA. Publication No. 89-1493, 264 pp.

Njau, R.J.A.; Mosha, F.W.; Nguma, J.F.M. 1993. Field trials of pyrethroid impregnated bednets in northern Tanzania. 1. Effect on malaria transmission. Insect Science and Its Applications, 5(6), 575–584.

Njunwa, K.J.; Lines, J.D.; Magesa, S.M.; Mnzava, A.E.P.; Wilkes, T.J.; Alilio, M.; Kivumbi, K.; Curtis, C.F. 1991. Trial of pyrethroid impregnated bednets in an area of Tanzania holoendemic for malaria. Part 1. Operation methods and acceptability. Acta Tropica, 49, 87–96.

PATH (Program for Appropriate Technology in Health). 1995. Feasibility study for increasing the availability of insecticide impregnated bednets for malaria control. PATH, Ottawa, ON, Canada. 21 pp.

Pickering, H. 1993. Report on a three week visit to suggest possible reasons for the apparent failure of insecticide impregnated bednets to reduce morbidity and mortality in Zone 5 (URD South Bank) of The Gambia. London School of Hygiene and Tropical Medicine, London, UK. 6 pp.

Pietra, Y.; Procacci, G.; Sabatinelli, G.; Kumlien, S.; Lamizana L.; Rotigliano, G. 1991. Impact de l'utilisation des rideaux imprégnés de perméthrine sur le paludisme dans une zone rurale de haute transmission au Burkina Faso. Bulletin de la Société de pathologie exotique, 84, 375–385.

Pleass, R.J.; Armstrong, J.R.M.; Curtis, C.F.; Jawara, M.; Lindsay, S.W. 1993. Comparison of permethrin treatments for bednets in The Gambia. Bulletin of Entomological Research, 83, 133–140.

Plestina, R. 1989. Human safety. Informal consultation on the use of impregnated bednets and other materials for disease vector control. World Health Organization, Geneva, Switzerland. 23 pp.

Port, G.R.; Boreham, P.F.L. 1982. The effect of bednets on feeding by *Anopheles gambiae*. Bulletin of Entomological Research, 72, 483–488.

Premji, Z.; Lubega, P.; Hamisi, Y.; Mchopa, E.; Minjas, J.; Checkley, W.; Shiff, C. 1995. Changes in malaria-associated morbidity in children using insecticide treated mosquito nets in the Bagamoyo District of coastal Tanzania. Tropical Medicine and Parasitology, 46, 147–153.

Procacci, P.G.; Lamizana, L.; Kumlien, S.; Habluetzel, A.; Rotigliano, G. 1991. Permethrin-impregnated curtains for malaria control. Transactions of the Royal Society of Tropical Medicine and Hygiene, 85, 181–185.

Ramakrishna, J.; Brieger, W.R.; Adeniyi, J.D. 1990. Treatment of malaria and febrile convulsions: an educational diagnosis of Yoruba beliefs. International Quarterly of Community Health Education, 9(4), 305–319.

Ranque, P.; Touré, Y.T.; Soula, G.; Le Du, Y.; Diallo, Y.; Traoré, O.; Duflo, B.; Balique, H. 1984. Étude expérimental sur l'utilisation de moustiquaires imprégnées de deltaméthrine dans la lutte contre le paludisme. Parassitologia, 26, 261–268.

Rasmuson, M.R.; Seidel, R.E.; Smith, W.A.; Booth, E.M. 1988. Communication for child survival. Academy for Educational Development, Washington, DC, USA. 24 pp.

Richards, F.O., Jr; Klein, R.E.; Zea Flores, R.; Weller, S.; Gatica, M.; Zeissig, R.; Sexton, J. 1993. Permethrin-impregnated bed nets for malaria control in northern Guatemala: epidemiological impact and community acceptance. American Journal of Tropical Medicine and Hygiene, 49(4), 410–418.

Robert, V.; Carnevale, P. 1991. Influence of deltamethrin treatment of bednets on malaria transmission in the Kou Valley, Burkina Faso. Bulletin of the World Health Organization, 69, 735–740.

Roberts, D.R.; Andre, R.G. 1994. Insecticide resistance issues in vector-borne disease control. American Journal of Tropical Medicine and Hygiene, 50(suppl.), 21–34.

Robey, B.; Piotrow, P.T.; Salter, C. 1994. Family planning lessons and challenges: making programs work. Population Information Program, Baltimore, MD, USA. Population Reports Series J, No. 40. 63 pp.

Rozendaal, J.A. 1989. Impregnated mosquito nets and curtains for self-protection and vector control. Tropical Diseases Bulletin, 86, R1–R41.

Rozendaal, J.A.; Voorham, J.; Van Hoof, J.P.M.; Oostburg, B.F.J. 1989. Efficacy of mosquito nets treated with permethrin in Surinam. Medical and Veterinary Entomology, 3, 353–365.

Schreck, C.E.; Self, L.S. 1985. Bed nets that kill mosquitoes. World Health Forum, 6, 342–344.

Service, M.W. 1993. Community participation in vector-borne disease control. Annals of Tropical Medicine and Parasitology, 87(3), 223–234.

Sexton, J.D. 1993. The logistics and maintenance issues involved in the use of impregnated mosquito nets as a malaria control measure. Presented at USAID Impregnated Mosquito Net Workshop, 11–13 May 1993. USAID, Washington, DC, USA. 5 pp.

———— 1994. Impregnated bednets for malaria control: biological success and social responsibility. American Journal of Tropical Medicine and Hygiene, 50(suppl.), 72–81.

Sexton, J.D.; Ruebush, T.K., II; Brandling-Bennett, A.D.; Breman, J.D.; Roberts, J.M.; Odera, J.S.; Were, J.B.O. 1990. Permethrin-impregnated curtains and bednets prevent malaria in western Kenya. American Journal of Tropical Medicine and Hygiene, 43(1), 11–18.

Sivananthan, T.; Townson, H.; Ward, S.A. 1992. A possible role for cytochrome P-450 enzymes in resistance of anophelines to pyrethroid insecticides (abstract). Transactions of the Royal Society of Tropical Medicine and Hygiene, 86, 346.

Sloof, R., ed. 1964. Observations on the effect of residual DDT house spraying on behaviour and mortality in species of the *A. punctulatus* group. AW Sythoff Editions, Leiden, Netherlands. 134 pp.

Smith, A.; Webley, D.J. 1969. A verandah-trap hut for studying the house-frequenting habits of mosquitoes and for assessing insecticides. III. The effect of DDT on behaviour and mortality. Bulletin of Entomological Research, 59, 33–46.

Snow, R.W. 1994. Progress report to WHO. A trial of insecticide-treated bed nets on the Kenyan coast. WHO–TDR, World Health Organization, Geneva, Switzerland. 22 pp.

Snow, R.W.; Lengeler, C.; de Savigny, D.; Cattani, C. 1995. Insecticide-treated bed nets in control of malaria in Africa. Lancet, 345, 1056–1057.

Snow, R.W.; Lindsay, S.W.; Hayes, R.J.; Greenwood, B.M. 1988. Permethrin-treated bednets (mosquito nets) prevent malaria in Gambian children. Transactions of the Royal Society of Tropical Medicine and Hygiene, 82, 838–842.

Snow, R.W.; Nevill, C.G.; Some, E.S.; Marsh, V.; Mbogo, C.N.M. 1993. WHO funded trial of insecticide-treated bed-nets in the reduction of childhood mortality on the Kenyan coast: Interim report on the pre-intervention year and delivery phase. WHO/TDR, World Health Organization, Geneva, Switzerland. 34 pp.

Snow, R.W.; Phillips, A.; Lindsay, S.W.; Greenwood, B.M. 1988. How best to treat bed nets with insecticide in the field. Transactions of the Royal Society of Tropical Medicine and Hygiene, 82, 647–648.

Snow, R.W.; Rowan, K.; Greenwood, B.M. 1987. A trial of permethrin-treated bed-nets in the prevention of malaria in Gambian children. Transactions of the Royal Society of Tropical Medicine and Hygiene, 81, 563–567.

Somboon, P. 1993. Forest malaria vectors in northwest Thailand and a trial of control with pyrethroid-treated bednets. University of London, London, UK. PhD thesis. 254 pp.

Stephens, C.; Masamu, E.C.; Kiama, M.G.; Keto, A.J.; Kinenekejo, M.; Ichimori, K.; Lines, J. 1995. Knowledge of mosquitoes in relation to public and private control activities in the cities of Dar es Salaam and Tanga, Tanzania. Bulletin of the World Health Organization, 73(1), 97–104.

Stich, A.H.R.; Maxwell, C.A.; Haji, A.A.; Haji, D.M.; Machano, A.Y.; Mussa, J.K.; Mattaelli, A.; Haji, H.; Curtis, C.F. 1994. Insecticide-impregnated bed nets reduce malaria transmission in rural Zanzibar. Transactions of the Royal Society of Tropical Medicine and Hygiene, 88, 150–154.

Tabashnik, B.E. 1990. Modelling and evaluation of resistance management tactics. In Roush, R.T.; Tabashnik, B.E., ed., Pesticide resistance in arthropods. Chapman and Hall, New York, NY, USA.

Taplin, D.; Meiking, T.L. 1990. Pyrethrins and pyrethroids in dermatology. Archives of Dermatology, 126, 213–221.

Taylor, C.E.; Georghiou, G.P. 1979. Suppression of insecticide resistance by alteration of gene dominance and migration. Journal of Economic Entomology, 72, 105–109.

Thomson, M.C.; d'Alessandro, U.; Bennett, S.; Connor, S.J.; Langerock, P.; Jawara, M.; Todd, J.; Greenwood, B.M. 1994. Malaria prevalence is inversely related to vector density in The Gambia, West Africa. Transactions of the Royal Society of Tropical Medicine and Hygiene, 88, 638–643.

Thomson, M.C.; Connor, S.J.; Bennett, S.; d'Alessandro U.; Milligan, P.; Aikins, M.K.; Langerock, P.; Jawara, M.; Greenwood, B.M. 1996. Geographical perspectives on bednet use and malaria transmission in The Gambia, West Africa. Social Science and Medicine. [In press]

Tincknell, R.C. 1985. Pesticide regulations. In Turnbull, G., ed., Occupational hazards of pesticide use. Taylor and Francis, London, UK. pp. 79–98.

Van Bortel, W.; Barutwanayo, M.; Delacollette, C.; Coosemans, M. 1996. Motivation à l'acquisition et à l'utilisation des moustiquaires imprégnées dans une zone à paludisme stable au Burundi. Tropical Medicine and International Health, 1(1), 71–80.

Vulule, J.M.; Beach, R.F.; Atieli, F.K.; Roberts, J.M.; Mount, D.L.; Mwangi, R.W. 1994. Reduced susceptibility of Anopheles gambiae to permethrin associated with the use of permethrin-impregnated bednets and curtains in Kenya. Medical and Veterinary Entomology, 8, 71–75.

Walsh, D.C.; Rudd, R.E.; Moeykens, B.A.; Moloney, T.W. 1993. Social marketing for public health. Health Affairs, 1993 (summer), 104–119.

WHO (World Health Organization). 1986a. Organophosphorus insecticides: a general introduction. WHO Environmental Health Criteria No. 63. 112 pp.

———— 1986b. Carbamate insecticides: a general introduction. WHO Environmental Health Criteria No. 64. 145 pp.

———— 1990a. Permethrin. WHO Environmental Health Criteria No. 94. 125 pp.

———— 1990b. Deltamethrin. WHO Environmental Health Criteria No. 97. 133 pp.

———— 1990c. Cyhalothrin. WHO Environmental Health Criteria No. 99. 106 pp.

———— 1990d. Cyhalothrin and lambdacyhalothrin health and safety guide. WHO Health and Safety Guide No. 38. 54 pp.

———— 1991. Safe use of pesticides. WHO Technical Report Series No. 813. 27 pp.

———— 1993a. Implementation of the global malaria control strategy. Report of a WHO study group on the implementation of the global plan of action for malaria control 1993–2000. WHO Technical Report Series No. 839. 57 pp.

———— 1993b. A global strategy for malaria control. WHO, Geneva, Switzerland. 30 pp.

———— 1994. World malaria situation in 1992. Weekly Epidemiological Record, 21 Oct 1994, 309–314.

WHO–VBC (World Health Organization – Village Bednet Committee). 1989. The use of impregnated bed-nets and other materials for vector-borne diseases. WHO, Geneva, Switzerland. WHO/VBC/89 No. 981 32 pp.

World Bank. 1993. World development report 1993: investing in health. Oxford University Press, New York, NY, USA. 329 pp.

Winch, P.J.; Kendall, C.; Gubler, D.J. 1992. Effectiveness of community participation in vector-borne disease control. Health Policy and Planning, 7(4), 342–351.

Winch, P.J.; Makemba, A.M. 1993. Plan of work for 1994. Bagamoyo Bed Net Project. Muhimbili Medical Centre, Dar es Salaam, Tanzania. 22 pp.

Winch, P.J.; Makemba, A.M.; Kamazima, S.R.; Lwihula, G.K.; Lubega, P.; Minjas, J.N.; Shiff, C.J. 1994. Seasonal variation in the perceived risk of malaria: implications for the promotion of insecticide-impregnated bed nets. Social Science and Medicine, 39, 63–75.

Winch, P.J.; Makemba, A.M.; Premji, Z.; Minjas, J.N.; Shiff, C.J. 1993. Operational issues in mosquito net interventions. Part 1: Factors affecting the demand for and usage of insecticide-impregnated mosquito nets. Paper presented at the USAID Impregnated Mosquito Net Workshop, 11–13 May 1993. USAID, Washington, DC, USA. 6 pp.

Xu, B.; Li, H.; Webber, R.H. 1994. Malaria in Hubei Province, China: approaching eradication. Journal of Tropical Medicine and Hygiene, 97, 277–281.

Zandu, A.; Malengreau, M.; Wery, M. 1991. Pratiques et dépenses pour la protection contre les moustiques dans les ménages à Kinshasa. Annales de la Société belge de médecine tropicale, 71, 259–266.

Ziba, C.; Slutsker, L.; Chitsulo, L.; Steketee, R.W. 1994. Use of malaria prevention measures in Malawian households. Tropical Medicine and Parasitology, 45, 70–73.

Zimicki, S.; Cham, K.; Greenwood, B.M. 1994. Report on the preliminary analyses of the 1994 national survey of knowledge, attitudes and practices
related to treatment of nets. National Impregnated Bednet Programme,
MRC Fajara, The Gambia. 33 pp.

Index